Dictionary of Disaster Medicine
and Humanitarian Relief

Dictionary of
Disaster Medicine
and Humanitarian Relief

Second Edition

By

S. William A. Gunn
MD, MS, FRCSC, FRCSI (Hon), DSc (Hon), Dr h c

President, International Association
for Humanitarian Medicine
President, International Federation of Surgical Colleges
President Emeritus, World Association
for Disaster and Emergency Medicine
Consultant to the United Nations

Formerly Head of Emergency Humanitarian Operations
World Health Organization

Foreword by the
Director-General Emeritus, World Health Organization

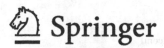 Springer

S. William A. Gunn
International Association for Humanitarian Medicine
La Panetière
Bogis-Bossey
Switzerland
swagunn@bluewin.ch

ISBN 978-1-4614-4444-2   ISBN 978-1-4614-4445-9 (eBook)
DOI 10.1007/978-1-4614-4445-9
Springer New York Heidelberg Dordrecht London

Library of Congress Control Number: 2012941618

Printed on acid-free paper

Springer is part of Springer Science+Business Media (www.springer.com)

This book is dedicated to

William H. Barton, OC, LLD
Canada's Ambassador to the United Nations,
distinguished diplomat, humanist and, above all,
friend

and to

all those who suffer from disasters
and those who bring relief in disasters

Foreword

If the Tower of Babel was a language disaster, disasters and humanitarian relief have their own language. Whether act of nature, act of man or folly of mankind, disasters are increasing alarmingly in frequency and magnitude, requiring an ever-growing complicated response from governments, organizations, specialists and humanitarian workers worldwide. Such major interventions are most often multidisciplinary, multilingual and of varied degrees of expertise, resulting in complications and unequal efficiency, with errors of communication, cooperation and action. In what is usually a difficult multisectoral field operation, the doctor must understand the engineer, the meteorologist must converse with the journalist, the nurse with the administrator, the ambulance man with the anaesthetist, the priest with the family, the WHO representative with the government and the coordinator with many NGOs from different cultures and countries. If such understanding is essential on the terrain, it is equally necessary away from the heat of action, at administrative tables, UN boardrooms, ministries, planning sessions, training courses, medical schools and philanthropic organizations, whence the need for a tool of common understanding, an essential standardized terminology as here presented.

I have known William Gunn over several decades and have particularly appreciated his productive work at the World Health Organization, where he was for many years head of Emergency Humanitarian Operations. Internationally acknowledged as a pioneer and innovator in disaster management, it may come as a surprise to many that he was also the Organization's chief of scientific terminology – surely an exceptional combination that has assured this remarkable book of special terminology, its authority and indispensable position. Indeed, its worth has been tested in numerous emergency interventions, operational tasks, organizational missions and editorial briefings within WHO, the UN, the Red Cross and many other national and international organizations since 1990, and this new expanded edition comes as a timely essential aid against the growing threats of inhuman violence and destructive disasters.

Director-General Emeritus
World Health Organization, Geneva

Halfdan Mahler, M.D.

History of this Book

Dictionary of Disaster Medicine and Humanitarian Relief
Second Edition
Springer Science, New York, 2013

Multilingual Dictionary of Disaster Medicine and International Relief
English, French, Spanish, Arabic
Kluwer Academic Publishers, Dordrecht, Boston, London, 1990
(Reprinted five times)

German edition: Wörterbuch der Katastrophenmedizin und der Internazionalen Hilfe
(with B. Domres, E. R. Steiner)
Stumpf and Kossendey, Edewecht, 1996

Japanese edition: Dictionary of Disaster Medicine and International Relief
(with M. Aono, T. Ukai, Y. Yamamoto)
Herusu Publishers, Tokyo, 1992

Civil Protection Multilingual Lexicon
(Commission of European Communities)
Eurodicautom Electronic Database, Brussels, 1991

Dictionnaire des Secours d'Urgence en cas de Catastrophe
(with C. Murcia, F. Parakatil)
CILF, Paris, 1984

Vocabulaire de l'Environnement
(with J. A. Ternisien, M. R. Amavis, et al.)
Hachette, Paris, 1976

History of this Book

About the Author

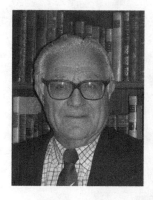

S. Wlliam A. Gunn, MD, MS, FRCSC, FRCSI (Hon), DSc (Hon), Dr.h.c., is a Canadian surgeon and senior international health scientist involved in emergency disaster management and humanitarian medicine. For many years he was director of the Emergency Humanitarian Operations of the World Health Organization, where he conducted numerous field missions, advised governments, the United Nations and the European Commission, organized high-level national programmes, lectured at universities and led training courses for disaster managers and humanitarian organizations, services that have been recognized by Honorary Doctorates and other high distinctions. Member of many surgical, emergency and humanitarian institutions, Dr. Gunn was a founder, now President Emeritus, of the World Association for Disaster and Emergency Medicine, founder of the WHO Medical Society and the International Association for Humanitarian Medicine, and life member of the Société Académique. He has been associated with many international bodies in a variety of senior capacities, inter alia as scientific coordinator of the European Centre for Disaster Medicine (Cross and ribbon of St. Agatha), honorary chair of the Asia-Pacific Conferences on Disaster Medicine, programme director of the International Civil Defence Organization, science terminologist to the Conseil International de la Langue Française, president of the International Federation of Surgical Colleges, foreign affairs advisor to the Red Cross Federation, consultant to the United Nations and medico-surgical expert to the Chair of the UN Fund for Torture Victims. Teacher and prolific writer, Professor Gunn is editor of several disaster and humanitarian journals and author of nineteen books. He has also been chief of WHO's scientific terminology, which further explains the high standard-setting lexicographic authority of his many specialized Dictionaries.

Introductory Note

This book is divided into two parts: Part I: Dictionary, and Part II: Acronyms and Abbreviations. The Dictionary constitutes the main body of the work, each entry being defined in detail, with synonyms and cross-references to other relevant terms. Part II defines an extensive list of acronyms and abbreviations that are commonly used in disaster medicine and international humanitarian relief.

The following abbreviations are used in the text:

Cf.   compare with or see the term mentioned
Sn: this term has a synonym, which is also defined
Sm: symbol
e.g. for example
*   this abbreviation is further defined in Part I

Some Press Comments on the First Edition

All those who are dealing with disaster relief work should have it.

The United Nations Disaster Relief Coordinator

Written by a pioneer in Disaster Medicine ...the Dictionary serves as an invaluable tool for the disaster manager. The entries clearly defined establish the standard vocabulary of disaster management and will be of great help to all those involved in emergency humanitarian endeavours.

The Ark, WHO Bulletin on Health Emergencies

The first compilation of all the technical terms and administrative abbreviations used in relief work.

Community Health Care, USA

Very useful document which all those who are dealing with disaster relief should have.

UNDRO News

This valuable book of reference has found a place of honour.

Corps Suisse d'Aide en cas de Catastrophe

The entire terminology of relief from A to Z explained in clear terms.

UNHCR, Refugiados / Refugees

Written by an acknowledged expert, solves a long-felt need. It establishes the standard terminology and should go a long way to improving the vital lines of communication in major emergency action and prevention.

International Civil Defence Journal

We welcome this most timely and remarkable multidisciplinary encyclopaedia. All the likely terms that may be encountered not only in the medical and humanitarian field but also in meteorology, administration, transport, geology, nuclear and conventional war and all other disaster situations, are clearly defined and constitute in fact the standard vocabulary ... Indespensable tool for all disaster managers, whatever their background and wherever they may be called upon to work: in the field, at the planning board, or just before setting out on a humanitarian mission. The only guide of its kind.

Annals of Burns and Fire Disasters

Work pioneered by SWA Gunn in the first attempt to gain understanding through standardization of the language and concepts we use in describing the greatest threats to humankind.

Prehospital and Disaster Medicine

Also by S. William A. Gunn

Health Sciences

Concepts and Practice of Humanitarian Medicine
(with M. Masellis)

Springer, New York, 2008

Chinese edition: Concepts and Practice of Humanitarian Medicine
(with Y-T. Wang)

Peoples' Medical Publishers, Beijing, 2011

Understanding the Global Dimensions of Health
(with P. Mansourian, A.M. Davies, A. Piel, B. McA. Sayers)

Springer, New York, 2005

Humanitarian Medicine
(with M. Masellis)

IAHM Publications, Palermo, 2005

The Management of Burns and Fire Disasters
(with M. Masellis)

Kluwer Academic Publishers, Dordrecht, London, Boston, 1995

The Management of Mass Burn Casualties and Fire Disasters
(with M. Masellis)

Kluwer Academic Publishers, Dordrecht, London, Boston, 1992

Health Technology Standards
(with N. J. O'Riordan)

ISO Publications, Geneva, 1991

Burns – Interactive Multimedia Hypertext CD-ROM
(with M. Costagliola, G. Magliacani, M. Masellis)

Informed, Palermo, 1989

Attacco alla Città
(with R. Clarke and GLAWARS Commission)

Edizioni Guida, Palermo, 1987

London Under Attack
(with R. Clarke and GLAWARS Commission)

Basil Blackwell Publishers, Oxford and New York, 1986

WHO Emergency Health Kit

World Health Organization, Geneva, 1984

Refugee Community Health Care
(with S. Simmonds and P. Vaughan)

Oxford University Press, Oxford, 1983 and 1985

Anthropology

Totem Poles of British Columbia Canada
(Reprinted seven times)

Macdonald and Whiterocks, Vancouver, 1965–1981

Acknowledgements

You cannot improve what you are unable to define.
C. Rollins Hanlon

Mal nommer les choses c'est ajouter au malheur du monde.
Albert Camus

Over approximately five decades, I have had the privilege of working, cooperating, discussing, arguing, collaborating, reading, comparing or dissecting words and in the process having fun, with a large number of persons, institutions, universities, researchers, writers, editors, journals, organizations, publishers, librarians, book lovers and wordsmiths, the expression of which constitutes this book, in second expanded edition. Some encounters have been extensive and professional, others light and occasional. They have been in the course of planned international negotiations or impromptu meetings, in sweltering disaster missions or comfortable academic boardrooms, profound discussions or neighbourly conversations, friendly journal clubs, scissors-and-paste reference sessions, literary divergences or obscure terminological explorations. All this is far from the methodical listing of bibliographies, meticulous alphabetical references and the usual "thank you" lines courteously added at the end of erudite articles. Whence the unorthodox mix, below, of authors, books, journals and organizations, acknowledged in an unusual way, but not without my warm appreciation of each one's invaluable contribution. And to forestall the inevitable missed out or absent name, let me respectfully add the more orthodox et al.

I thank the Academic Council on the United Nations System, Jakov Adler, the American Medical Writers' Association, Sadruddin Aga Khan, John Agad, Naoki Aikawa, Ali Al Numairy, All Russian Zashchita, Eric Alley, *Annals of Burns and Fire Disasters*, *Annales de Droit International Médical*, Makoto Aono, Jeffrey Arnold, Gösta Arturson, Yasufumi Asai, Jo Asvall, Bishara Atiyeh, Jan Babik, Ibrahim Badran, Zbigniew Bankowski, the BASICS group, *Basics of International Humanitarian Missions*, Peter Baskett, Fabrizio Bassani, Peter Baxter, Henrick

Beer, Yves Beigbeder, Michel Bélanger, Fortunato Benaim, Farouk Berkol, Rosalie Bertell, Marvin Birnbaum, Richard Bissell, Bradford University Disaster Prevention and Limitation Unit, *British Columbia Medical Journal*, *British Medical Journal*, Frederick Burkle Jr., *Butterworths Medical Dictionary*, Kevin Cahill, Canadian Medical Association and its *Journal*, Pierre Carli, Luciano Carrino, University of Louvain Centre for Research in the Epidemiology of Disasters, Leonardo Cenci, Centre Europe-Tiers Monde, Howard Champion, CIOMS, Robin Clarke, *the Concise Oxford Dictionary*, Victor Condé, Conseil International de la Langue Française, Michel Costagliola, Dag Hammerskjöld Library, Michel Debacker, Jan De Boer, *Définitions des Droits de l'Homme*, Herman Delooz, Flavio Del Ponte, *Dictionary of Public Health*, DERC, *Disaster Management Glossary*, Delft University, Claude De Ville De Goyet, *DHA News*, Wolfgang Dick, Disaster Research Center at Delaware University, *Disaster Prevention and Management*, Oksana Dmitrienko, Giovanni Dogo, Bernd Domres, Russell Dynes, Jan Egeland, Anne Ehrlich, Olavi Elo, M'Hamed Essaafi, European Centre for Disaster Medicine, EU *Civil Protection Multilingual Lexicon*, FAO *Wildland Fire Management Terminology*, William Feindel, Alain Flaujat, Jean Marie Fonrouge, Fordham University Center for International Health and Cooperation, Robert Fortuine, *From Sarajevo to Hiroshima*, Giovanni Galassi, William C. Gibson, Sergei Goncharov, Kyoko Goto, Graduate Institute of Geneva, Wayne Greene, Brian Gushulak, C. Rollins Hanlon, Yoshikura Haraguchi, EC *Health and Human Rights*, Herusu Tokyo Publications, Kendall Ho, Jean-Pierre Hocké, Edgar Housepian, Norman Howard-Jones, Hradec Kràlové Faculty of Military Health Sciences, Zi-Tong Huang, Pierre Huguenard, HCHR *Human Rights – Compilation of International Instruments*, *Humanitarian Initiative Against "Political Disappearances"*, IDNDR *International Glossary of Disaster Management*, International Association for Humanitarian Medicine, International Civil Defence Organization, *International Review of the Red Cross*, International Federation of Surgical Colleges, *International Humanitarian Assistance – Disaster Relief Actions in International Law and Organization*, International Institute of Humanitarian Law, Institut Henry Dunant, *International Human Rights Lexicon*, *JAMA*, Jiang Jian, *Journal of Humanitarian Medicine*, Vit Karnik, A.Z.Keller, Leo Klein, Kluwer Academic Publishers, Mark Klyachko, Radana Königova, Joachim Kreysler, Per Kulling, Adam Kushner, Tore Laerdal, Robert H. Lane, John M. Last, Michel Lechat, League (now Federation) of Red Cross and Red Crescent Societies, Zhongmin Liu, Alessandro Loretti, Norberto Liwski, London School of Hygiene and Tropical Medicine, Timothy Lusty, Corrado Manni, Pierre Mansourian, Michele Masellis, Matti Mattila, Sophocles Mavrantonis, *The Medical Implications of Nuclear War*, *Medicus Mundi*, Meneghetti Foundation, Jacques Meurant, Hanifa Mezoui, *Multilingual Dictionary of Disaster Medicine and International Relief*, Natural Hazards Center University of Colorado, B. Nemitz, Krisno Nimpuno, Norifumi Ninomiya, Eric Noji, Karl-Axel Norberg, Helena Nygren-Krug, UN Office for the Coordination of Humanitarian Affairs (previously UNDRO), Muneo Ohta, *On Better Terms – A UN Glance at Key Climate Change and Disaster Risk Reduction Concepts*, Osler Library, Chander Parkash, *Origins*, Jovica Patrnogic, the *Penguin Atlas of Diasporas*, Pierre Perrin, Nelson Piccolo,

Jean Pictet, Anthony Piel, Pittsburg University Center for Resuscitation Research, Jiri Pokorny, *Prehospital and Disaster Medicine, Printing and the Mind of Man*, Basil Pruitt Jr., Pugwash Conferences on Science and World Affairs, Demetrios Pyrros, E.L.Quarantelli, *Questions d'Ethique Soulevées par la Biotechnologie*, Abdul Radjak, *Refugee Survey Quarterly, Report of the Greater London Area War Risk Study*, Norman Rich, Rockefeller Library and Museum, Gerald Rockenschaub, Leonid Roshal, Joseph Rotblat, Royal College of Surgeons of England, Royal College of Surgeons in Ireland, Royal College of Physicians and Surgeons of Canada, Lu Rushan, Rémi Russbach, Peter Safar, Ritsuro Sakurai, John Schou, Debarati Guha-Sapir, Genevieve Schweizer, *The Secret Life of Words*, Sergey Shoigu, Martin Silverstein, Robert Souria, Knut Ole Sundnes, Stockholm International Peace Research Institute, Task Force on Quality Control of Disaster Management, Haroun Tazieff, *The Words of Medicine – Sources, Meanings and Delights*, Marija Trop, Takashi Ukai, *The Lancet*, UNDRO Disaster Management Terms, *UNDRO News, UN Chronicle, UN Human Rights System, UNISDR Terminology on Disaster Risk Reduction*, Adriaan Van Es, Theo van Boven, Michel Veuthey, Cedric Viale, *A Voice for Human Rights, Voluntary Work in Society Today*, Jaap Walkate, Yi-Tang Wang, Henry Wilson, the WHO and UN Libraries, WHOPAX Advisory Board, *Wordsworth Dictionary of Science and Technology, World Journal of Surgery*, WMA *Medical Ethics Manual*, Shao Xiaohong, Yasuhiro Yamamoto, G. Zamberletti and numerous reports, records, documents, terminology banks, journals, guides, books and other publications of the World Health Organization and the United Nations System, where this book saw its beginnings.

I owe a separate section and special thanks to Yves Schweizer, without whose patience and computer expertise this manuscript would still remain an MS, to Jean Gunn for her meticulous editing, to Bill Tucker and Khristine Queja of Springer Publishers for their professional guidance, and of course to Dr Halfdan Mahler for his generous Foreword and particularly for the privilege of working with him for many years for a humanitarian cause against disasters and for human well-being.

Bogis-Bossey   S. William A. Gunn
Switzerland

Contents

Contents

Part I
Dictionary

A

Abandon To give up or forsake. To break off a relationship of dependency, as between parent and child.
Cf. unaccompanied minor

Abate To mitigate violence, to lower a risk, to weaken in force or intensity, to reduce, to attenuate.
Cf. attenuation

ABCDE Mnemonic acronym for Airway, Breathing, Circulation, Disability, Exposure. A primary extended but rapid survey in case of grave multiple injury to be performed in no more than 2–5 min.
Cf. ABC, AVPU

Abduct Anatomy: To move a limb laterally, away from the midline.
Law: To carry away illegally; to separate forcefully; to kidnap.
Cf. kidnap, deport

Abnormal A state or quality of being outside the established parameters or of deviating from the usually accepted norm. A malformation.

Abolitionism Doing away with, terminating totally. In the eighteenth and nineteenth centuries, it referred mainly to the social movement and objective of ending black peoples' slavery. Currently, it mainly aims at abolishing the death penalty and terminating other inequalities and injustices in human rights.

A-bomb Sn: atom bomb, atomic bomb
Cf. nuclear war, weapon of mass destruction

Aborigine The indigenous or original living people (and fauna and flora) of a particular geographical region, before the arrival of colonists.
In Australia and Canada, the designation of the original people of these countries. In Canada also called First Nations.
Cf. absorption, acculturation, ethnic group, racial discrimination

Abort Medicine: Premature delivery of a child. Miscarry.
Firefighting: To jettison a load of water or retardant from an aircraft – FAO.
Management: To terminate prematurely an unsuccessful project or action.

Abortion, unsafe The termination of an unintended pregnancy either by persons lacking the necessary skills or in an environment lacking the minimal medical standards, or both. The brunt of unsafe abortions occurs primarily in the developing world – WHO.

S.W.A. Gunn, *Dictionary of Disaster Medicine and Humanitarian Relief*,
DOI 10.1007/978-1-4614-4445-9_1, © Springer Science+Business Media New York 2013

Absolute (human) right A right that exists at all times, stays asserted under all circumstances, cannot be restricted or derogated. Example: freedom from torture – after V. Condé. Cf. Universal Declaration of Human Rights, rights – inalienable

Absorbed dose The quantity of a substance (drug, pollutant) or energy (ionizing radiation) received during a given time by a person, group or environment.
Cf. ionizing radiation, nuclear energy, pollutant, retained dose, gray (Gy units)

Absorption Social: The process by which an individual is assimilated by a community, system or society, resulting in changes in the absorbed individual but not in the absorbing system. Example: cultural absorption. Cf. acculturation, assimilation
Biology: Transformation of a nutrient, drug or pollutant, into cellular material by a living organism.
Hydrology: Sucking in of fluid.

Abuja Declaration Solemn undertaking in 2001 of African leaders pledging to "set a target of at least 15% of their annual budgets for the improvement of the health sector" – WHO.
Cf. Paris Declaration, Accra Agenda

Abuse Health: The excessive, wrong or improper use of health-care services or products, such as drugs.
General: Misuse, treat badly by committing improper action, or by omitting necessary action.

Academic Council on the United Nations System/ACUNS: A highly professional association of educational and research institutions and individual scholars, teachers, academics, politologues and practitioners active in multilateral relations, world politics, global governance, UN-related issues and international cooperation.
Sn: ACUNS

Acaricide Sn: miticide

Acceleration The rate of change in velocity in a given time. In seismology, the variation in the movement of a point on the earth or of a structure during an earthquake. It is expressed as a fraction of gravity and is measured by the accelerograph.
Cf. earthquake, seismograph

Acceptable collateral damage: In military operations, a degree of unintended damage that is subjectively considered the victim could accept or live with, as part of the unfortunate and unavoidable price of achieving the military objective.
Cf. collateral damage

Acceptable risk The eventual loss and agreed conditions or degree of human, material and economic damage that a country or community is willing to accept as tolerable under the prevailing economic, social, political, technical, structural and other conditions, rather than provide the necessary finances, efforts and resources to reduce such a risk.
Cf. disaster act, disaster preparedness, disaster probability, risk

Access: health care/security Health: Access to health care is a human right, and patients must be provided with the necessary facilities to reach or to obtain the needed health care. Access may be influenced by (a) the availability of health personnel, transport and infrastructures, (b) by patient-related factors and (c) at the structural level, by the organization of health systems.

Security: Persecution victims must have access to advice, comfort assistance and necessary protection.

Accident/Incident Accident, a sudden, unforeseen event that can cause varying degrees of harm and/or destruction, from mild damage to serious injury or death. It is more serious than incident, although these two terms are often misused interchangeably in emergency management. Accident requires greater attention and response, whence accident prevention, accident departments in hospitals, accident legislation, emergency services.
Cf. incident/accident, chemical accident, emergency

Accident site In disaster medicine, the place where the rescue team is in operation to extricate and relieve the victims – EU.

Acclimatization Adjustment of a living organism to a new climatic environment other than that to which it has been accustomed. By extension, it is also used for non-climatic adjustment.

Accountability Liability of persons, groups or governments to be called to account, to be answerable before the law for decisions and actions that they have undertaken and are responsible to maintain, as agreed. (The opposite would be impunity.)
Cf. Vienna Declaration, impunity

Accra Agenda for Action In the field of health financing, a call, in 2008, to donor countries to strengthen their commitments for national health planning and improvement in support of the Millennium Development Goals.
Cf. Paris Declaration, Abuja Declaration, Millennium Development Goals

Acculturation Process by which a human society assimilates or adopts part or all of the customs, beliefs and cultural values of another society. Also refers to the results of such assimilation.
Cf. absorption, assimilation

Acetone peroxide, TAPT A chemical explosive of artisanal manufacture often used in suicide bombing and terrorist attacks. Easily available ingredients are hydrogen peroxide, acetone and sulphuric or hydrochloric acid. Also known as TAPT or Mother of Satan.
Sn: TAPT

Acid rain Sulphuric acid (H_2SO_4) in the atmosphere, formed by the combination of sulphur trioxide with water, resulting in a relatively stable mist of acid droplets. In excessive concentrations in the air, it increases the acidity of the soil and disturbs the pH causing agricultural and ecological damage.
Cf. air pollution, transboundary pollution

Acquired immunodeficiency syndrome/AIDS A highly infectious disease of pandemic proportions, caused by the HIV virus. Also referred to as HIV/AIDS. A person who has the virus is a carrier and can infect others. Spread is by sexual intercourse, by contaminated needles and syringes, transfusion of infected blood, by body fluids, by infected mother to her unborn child. Spread is unlikely through daily social contact, such as shaking hands.
Note: Non-infective immune deficiency can also be acquired through radiation.
Sn: AIDS, HIV/AIDS
Cf. HIV, immunodeficiency

Action phase/of disaster Within the varying stages of disaster management, the actual direct action emergency response phase. In all preparedness programmes and especially to face emergencies that may occur without warning, it is essential to have an established plan for action.
Cf. phases of disaster, action plan

Action plan A tactical plan developed by the competent directorate, the emergency team or the incident command system, in support of the organization's projected progress, or of successfully managing the emergency, or of the incident action strategy against a specific disaster.
Cf. disaster management

Active volcano A volcano that is known to have erupted in the past and which, although silent or non-eruptive at the present time, can be expected to erupt at an indeterminate time, as based on oral tradition, archives and scientific observations.
Cf. volcanic risk map

Activity (nuclear) The spontaneous emission of alpha, beta or sometimes gamma rays from the disintegration of the nuclei of atoms per second. The unit of radioactivity is the becquerel (Bq).
Cf. becquerel, nuclide, radioactivity, nuclear activity

Acute/Chronic Health Evaluation – APACHE scale Medicine: Acute physiology and chronic health evaluation: APACHE. A numerical score to predict patient outcomes, performance and prognosis, in seriously ill patients. Ethnology: A major indigenous tribe of North America.

Acute radiation syndrome Cf. radiation sickness

Acute respiratory disease Term that refers to several acute, mild to severe infections of the respiratory tract, caused by a variety of viruses and bacteria. It ranges from the common cold to influenza, bronchitis, even to fatal pneumonia and SARS. A major cause of illness and mortality in disaster situations.
Cf. infection, severe acute respiratory syndrome

Adaptation The process and the result of physical, biological and psychological changes of an organism or a population in order to adjust to given environmental conditions.
Cf. degree of adaptability, environment, coping, society, adjustment

Adaptive capacity The ability of living organisms to respond to changes of different nature and adjust to actual or expected variations, thus coping with situations and increasing their chances of survival and well-being.
Cf. coping

Addict/Addiction A person who has the unsocial behaviour of dependence on a drug or toxic substance which, when discontinued, can aggravate the situation with additional pathological withdrawal effects.
Addiction is the state of such dependence, substance dependence.
Cf. dependence, drug

Adequacy A health programme or action is adequate if it is proportionate to requirements – HFA.

Adjustment Adapting, reconciling, modifying differences both at the human, behavioural level, such as on arrival into a new society, and at the physical, external level, such as altering office space to accommodate new work.
Cf. adaptation

Adobe Mud brick that is only sun-dried but not burned or kilned. Extensively used in developing countries for low-cost housing, particularly vulnerable in earthquakes and floods.

Advanced life support/Advanced trauma life support In a critically ill patient, after ensuring basic life support, the further (= advanced) resuscitative measures taken by trained personnel, such as life-saving medication, electrocardiography and heart defibrillation, to restore spontaneous blood circulation and resuscitation and to avert death.
Sn: ALS; ATLS
Cf. basic life support, cardiopulmonary resuscitation, Glasgow trauma scale

Advective thunderstorm Thunderstorm arising from the instability produced by the advection of cold air in the upper levels, or of warm air at lower levels, or by the combination of both.

Adverse medical/drug event Medical: An injury that is caused by medical management rather than by underlying disease and that prolongs hospitalization, produces disability at discharge or both – Inst. Med. US.
Drug: An event that is noxious, unintended and occurs at doses used in man for prophylaxis, diagnosis, therapy or modification of functions – WHO.

Advocacy Pleading, arguing, favouring, supporting and persuading for a worthy cause, policy, ideal, people, etc.

Affirmative action A sociolegal concept introduced in the United States to take positive measures to redress certain existing disadvantages by providing corrective favourable obligations, e.g. ensuring positive consideration to a black employee in respect of a competing white employee.

Afforestation The policy and process of establishing a forest in a previously non-forested area.
Cf. reforestation, deforestation, forestation

Aflatoxins Carcinogenic fungal toxins that can contaminate large quantities of corn, peanuts and other crops, causing widespread health risks. The Codex Alimentarius has set concentration limitations.

African trypanosomiasis Cf. trypanosomiasis, sleeping sickness, American trypanosomiasis, neglected tropical disease

Aftershock One or more smaller earth tremors that follow the main seismic shock and originate at or near the larger earthquake's epicentre. Foreshocks are the opposite, preceding the earthquake.
Cf. earthquake, epicentre, foreshock

Aga Khan Foundation International foundation that without discrimination promotes health, education, rural development, inter-religious relations and enhancement of relevant NGOs, especially in developing countries.
Cf. development, rural development

Age groups On the basis of health-relevant issues, life-span years are subdivided and named by categories that can vary according to country and legislation. Generally accepted groups are as follows:
Early childhood: from birth to 9 years
Child: up to age 18 years (UN). Also minor, juvenile
Adolescent: 10–19 years
Youth: 15–24 years
Adulthood: 20–59 years (including reproductive years 15–44)
Old age: 60 years and over
Cf. child

Age profile Graphic representation of the statistical composition of a population, during a given period, by the juxtaposition of histograms representing the age distribution by sex.
Also age pyramid.

Agent BZ A psychochemical of secret chemical structure developed as an incapacitating agent for chemical warfare.
Cf. chemical weapons

Agent G Represents a class of nerve gases used as chemical weapons. Highly toxic.
Cf. nerve gas, agent V, Geneva Protocol, chemical weapons

Agent orange A highly toxic herbicide (2,4,5,-T, trichlorophenoxyacetic acid) containing a high proportion of dioxin, used in military attacks over Vietnam, with great damage to vegetation and the population.
Cf. dioxin, Seveso, UN hazard classification

Agent V One of the nerve gases used as toxic chemical weapon.
Cf. nerve gas, agent G

Agent VX A highly toxic nerve gas, more lethal than sarin as a weapon.
Cf. sarin, nerve gas, chemical weapons

Aggression Illegal attack and criminal hostilities by a State against the independence and sovereignty of another.
According to the Nuremberg Court, "to initiate a war of aggression is not only an international crime, it is the supreme international crime". It is now considered a crime against peace.

Aggression, Crime of The UN General Assembly (Res.3314, xxix,1974) defined aggression as "the gravest and most dangerous form of unlawful use of force". The UN Charter not only prohibits the recourse to force but also the aggressive menace of using force, as being incompatible with the principles of the United Nations.
Cf. aggressiveness, Kampala Conference, Briand-Kellogg Pact

Aggressiveness A hostile position, act or threat, usually unprovoked, to establish dominance, induce fear or to protect territory, the family group or offspring.

Aid Free material or financial assistance or other support given to a needy organization, community or country, without expecting any gain.
Sn: assistance, relief, help
Cf. donor, humanitarian medicine, Paris Declaration

AIDS/Aids Acronymic term given to acquired immunodeficiency syndrome. Usually written in capital letters, less often as Aids. Caused by the HIV virus. Commonly referred to as HIV/AIDS.
Sn: acquired immunodeficiency syndrome
Cf. immunodeficiency, HIV virus

Air mass thunderstorm Thunderstorm which arises within an unstable air mass and which is not caused by the passage of a front.
Cf. thunderstorm

Air pollution Presence of considerable quantities of gaseous, liquid or solid contaminants in the atmosphere and liable to be harmful to animal, vegetable and human life.
Cf. atmosphere, pollutant, contamination, atmospheric pollution

ALARA/Alara Acronymic term for "As low as reasonably achievable", concerning the extent of needed interventions against the release of nuclear, chemical or other dangerous materials.

Alarm A visual, acoustic, semaphoric, radio or other emergency signal informing the population of an imminent danger and calling the relevant personnel to proceed to their appropriate responsibilities.
Cf. alert, warning

Alert An advisory signal notifying that a hazard is approaching. It is less imminent than an "alarm" or a "warning" signal.
Cf. epidemic alerts, WHO alerting degrees, alarm, warning

Algorithm A structured graphical process and representation of a systematic and logical sequence of interdependent steps to guide in decision-making, with the aim of arriving at optimal decisions.

Alien Any individual who is not a national of the State in which he or she is present – OHCHR.

Allergen Any substance such as pollen, toxin, drug or food that can act as an antigen and induce an allergic reaction in an organism.
Cf. allergy, antigen, immunization

Allergy The hyper-reaction or pathological response of a person or certain organisms to a given allergen.
Cf. allergen

Alleviate To lighten the burden, to relieve the suffering, to mitigate.
Cf. mitigate

Alluvium Debris, soil and particles resulting from erosion transported and deposited by a stream or by the sea.
Sn: alluvial deposit

Alma-Ata Declaration On September 12, 1978, at Alma-Ata, then in the Soviet Union, the World Health Organization, all its members and UNICEF unanimously signed the Declaration on Primary Health Care, which has become the global spearhead for the protection and promotion of all peoples' health and the foundation of the concept of Health For All.
Cf. primary health care, Health for All

Alternative technology Technology that, as an alternative to resource-intensive and wasteful industry, aims to utilize resources sparingly, with minimum damage to the environment, at affordable cost and with a possible degree of control over the processes.
Cf. TCDC, appropriate technology, sustainable development, MDGs

Altruism Regard and unselfish consideration of others, humanitarian concern for the welfare of the needy, with willingness to help as a principle.
Cf. humanitarian medicine, voluntary agency, pro bono

Amelisap Acronymic term for Association des Médecins Libéraux Sapeurs-Pompiers. French association of volunteer physicians trained for and active in forest fires, burns and disasters.
Cf. forest fires

American College of Surgeons Largest and most prestigious professional organization of surgeons, devoted to the study, teaching, practice and ethics of surgery nationally and internationally. Has a special programme "Operation Giving Back" and awards for volunteerism and humanitarian work to strengthen surgery in the developing countries.
Cf. Royal College of Surgeons of Canada, essential surgery, humanitarian surgery

American trypanosomiasis Sn: Chagas disease
Cf. African trypanosomiasis, neglected tropical disease

Amnesia Partial or complete loss of memory. Frequent in various degrees after a head injury or major accident.

Amnesty An expression of goodwill, offering general pardon, reconciliation on humane grounds, while remaining uncompromising on breaches of human rights.
Cf. Amnesty International

Amnesty International/AI An entirely independent and active international humanitarian movement that struggles for the liberation of prisoners of conscience, exposes breaches of human rights such as torture, disappearances, hostage taking, impunity and renders the world conscious of such persecutions. Respected and valuable actions that earned AI the Nobel Peace Prize in 1977.
Cf. amnesty, human rights, disappearances, prisoners of conscience, torture

Amoebiasis A parasitic disease of the intestinal tract due to *Entamoeba histolytica* dysentery with occasionally liver complications. It is associated with hot climates, poor sanitation and faecal contamination of water. Disaster conditions, with overcrowding, increase the spread of amoebiasis. Also amebiasis.
Cf. dysentery, enteric diseases

Amplitude tidal range The difference between the height of the mean level and the maximum or minimum height of the water in the partial movement caused by the wave.
Sn: tidal range
Cf. tide, tidal scale

Anaemia Diminution of the quantity of red cells and functional haemoglobin of the blood, which may be due to multiple causes: malaria, haemolysis, sickle cell anaemia, hookworms, bleeding, iron and other nutritional deficiencies. Widespread. A major problem in pregnant women.
Also anemia.

Anarchism From the Greek an = without, and archos = rule, the belief that society does not need rules or an organized State to function, which is considered harmful and must be abolished.

Anchor point In firefighting, an advantageous point of a barrier from which a protective fire line can be constructed, especially to reduce the hazard of being outflanked by the flames.

Angst Marked anxiety, despair, feeling of gloom. Common in disaster situations and in face of injustice.

Animism A belief that objects, phenomena and happenings in nature, such as trees, gales, earthquakes, have a spirit, totem and conscious life. In some cultures and primitive beliefs, animism is used to explain natural disasters, catastrophes, disease, healing and other phenomena.
Cf. natural disaster, traditional medicine, shamanism, totem.

Ankylostomiasis A debilitating parasitic disease of the intestinal tract caused by two kinds of hookworm, especially prevalent in tropical and subtropical areas. Gives pharyngeal and laryngeal manifestations and a major cause of anaemia. Spread by plantar exposure, it can be individually prevented by wearing shoes.
Cf. enteric diseases

Annual flood The annual peak discharge of water observed in one year.

Answerable The liability of a person, community or state called to account; responsible for acts committed.

Antenatal Before birth; during gestation. Special clinics are conducted for
the care of expectant mothers. Mother
and child are particularly at risk in
situations of disaster and poverty.
Sn: prenatal

Anthrax A contagious disease of animals caused by *Bacillus anthracis*,
infrequently transmitted to man
through contact, ingestion or inhalation. Infection renders immunity. Has
been used as a biological weapon for
terrorist purposes.
Cf. zoonosis, biological warfare,
bioterrorism

Anthropic erosion Man-made land
erosion caused or accelerated by
excessive clearing or grazing, with
destruction of the surface vegetation,
which leads to the degradation of the
upper layers of the soil.
Cf. man-made disaster, erosion,
desertification

Antiballistic missile A military pilotless rocket-propelled projectile
(missile) designed to intercept and
destroy an incoming enemy ballistic
missile or its warhead before it
reaches its target. The antiballistic
missile defence (ABM) Treaty of
1972 limited the deployment of
antiballistic missiles and restricted
their development. It distinguished
between "strategic" or long-range
missiles (prohibited) and "non-strategic" or short-range missiles (not
prohibited). This Treaty terminated
in 2002 when the Strategic Offensive
Reduction Treaty (SORT) came into
force. To be reviewed in 2012.
Sn: ABM
Cf. strategic defence initiative, arms
race, ballistic missile, star wars, SALT,
START

Antibody An immunoglobulin serum
protein in the body that binds with a
specific antigen and confers protection against it.
Cf. antigen, vaccination

Anticyclone An atmospheric zone of
relatively high pressure, normally
characterized by fine weather and
freak winds. It circulates clockwise
in the northern and counterclockwise
in the southern hemisphere.
Cf. cyclone, atmospheric pressure,
wind

Antidote A chemical or medicine given
to counter a specific poisoning.

Antigen Biological substance in the
blood capable of stimulating the
formation of protective antibodies.
Cf. antibody, vaccination

Antimissile shield A much disputed
defensive/offensive plan of the United
States envisaging the placement of a
belt of long-range antimissile weaponry along the eastern borders of
Europe.
Cf. star wars, START-II

Apartheid An Afrikaans term introduced in 1929 to signify the separation of the black population of South
Africa from the supposedly superior
white population, based on the illegal
and immoral racist concepts of
supremacy, resulting in unlawful segregation, injustices, persecution and
pauperization of the black people.
Abolished after the fall of the
undemocratic racist regime.
Cf. racism, segregation, human rights

Apathy Absence of concern, indifference, lack of motivation. Such a temporary passive attitude is not rare
among disaster victims. It can also be
observed in groups for various
reasons.

Apatride French word, from a/patrie, meaning "without a fatherland", a stateless person.
Cf. stateless, refugee

Appeal Emergency: A request by a governmental or non-governmental organization to a government or the public for financial support to a charitable or humanitarian cause, or to counter a disaster.
Cf. declaration of disaster
Legal: Appeals court: a higher court that re-examines cases previously tried in an inferior court.

Appropriate technology Techniques, knowledge, methods, procedures and equipment that are adapted and appropriate to local needs, acceptable to those who use them and to those for whom they are used, scientifically valid yet uncomplicated, which can be maintained and utilized with the resources the country or community can afford.
Cf. alternative technology, technology transfer, TCDC

Aquiculture The production of aquatic plants or animals in a marine or fresh water environment for commercial purposes.
Sn: aquaculture

Arbitration The binding settlement of a political, social or industrial dispute by the decision of a mutually agreed or chosen one-time arbitral tribunal or conciliator called for that purpose.

Archipelago A group of islands. Example: the Archipelago of Azores

Ariboflavinosis Sn: vitamin B_2 deficiency

Arid A climate or land in which the humidity and rainfall are insufficient to counterbalance the evaporation and loss of water necessary for vegetation.
Cf. desert, semi-arid zone

Aridity Characteristic of a climate where precipitation is insufficient to maintain vegetation.
Cf. arid, semi-arid zone

Arithmetic growth Growth of an organism or population by linear increase in size or number.
Cf. exponential growth

Armed conflict War. A state of hostilities in which two or more organized armies are at war against each other. In modern warfare, the attack may be with conventional arms, chemical and/or biological weapons or nuclear weapons.
Cf. Geneva Conventions, CBW, atomic bomb, biological warfare, chemical warfare

Arms control Measures taken by a State – or required by the United Nations – intended to limit or reduce forces, regulate armaments and restrict the deployment of troops or weapons, with the view to rendering that State less dangerous and to inducing similar behaviour in other State(s), pursuant to an agreement.
Cf. disarmament

Arms race Since the end of the Cold War, the arms race has slackened but not ended. The military capacity of three major nations at mid-2011 is as follows: Nuclear warheads: US 8,500, Russia 11,000, China 240; Military personnel: US 1,560,000, Russia 1,050,000, China 2,290,000; Submarines: US 71, Russia 67, China 71; Warships: US 112, Russia 31, China 78; Aircraft carriers: US 11, Russia 1, China 0; Combat aircraft: US 3,897, Russia 1,880, China 1,998; Military spending (2010): US $698 billion, Russia $58.7 bn, China $119 bn – after SIPRI, IISS, *Time*.

Arsenalization of space The increasing use of the earth's atmosphere for military purposes with missiles, satellites, probes, space stations, etc. and resulting space débris.
Sn: militarization of space
Cf. strategic defence initiative, space race

Arson Criminal setting on fire of another's property or the intentional burning of one's own property when insured. A fire also set by an unstable individual for personal, psychopathological satisfaction.

Artificial feeding Infant feeding with milk other than human breast milk.

Ascariasis A parasitic infection of the intestine, frequent and sometimes endemic especially in children, in tropical countries. Caused by a nematode worm. Commonly transmitted through ingestion of food contaminated by faeces.
Cf. enteric diseases

Aseismic construction Design, building, rebuilding or retrofitting of any construction, such as houses, factories, bridges, dams, skyscrapers, hospitals, according to materials, mathematics and regulations destined to make the structure withstand collapse or damage during an earthquake.
Sn: antiseismic, nonseismic
Cf. Mercalli scale, Richter scale

Ash Fire: The residual content of a product after complete combustion.
Volcanology: Tiny fragments projected by a volcanic eruption.
Cf. tephra, ash flow, volcano

Ash fall The falling down of volcanic ash onto the ground after it has been projected into the air. The ash clouds following the Iceland volcanic erup-

tion in 2010 caused severe disruption of aviation and of agriculture.
Cf. ash

Ash flow In volcanic eruptions, most of the gas-charged ash remains close to the ground and falls by gravity like foam. It is a form of nuée ardente. Can cause severe respiratory distress.
Cf. ash, lahar, tephra, nuée ardente, volcano

Asia-Pacific Conferences on Disaster Medicine International professional group that studies, advises and promotes humanitarian health issues and emergency preparedness in the circum-Pacific countries which are highly disaster prone. Holds specialized conferences every two years, while its national counterparts, like the Japan Medical Team for Disaster Relief, are actively operational.
Cf. disaster medicine, international assistance, Japan Medical Team for Disaster Relief

Asphyxia Acute respiratory obstruction of airflow, with impairment of the oxygen supply to tissues due to reduced oxygen intake in the lungs, leading to imminent cell death.
Cf. respiratory distress

Assessment (of disaster) Survey of real or potential disaster to estimate the actual or expected damages and to make recommendations for preparedness, mitigation and relief action.
Cf. damage assessment, rapid assessment protocol

Assimilation
1. Biological: Transformation of nutrients into cellular material by a living organism.
2. Social: Cf. absorption

Assistance/Aid Providing help, relief and support with the aim of diminishing a person's or community's suffering or increasing their capacity to cope. Such material and social assistance and humane aid are primordial in disaster situations and are provided by individuals, governments and humanitarian volunteer bodies.
Cf. relief, humanitarian medicine, voluntary associations, aid

Association for Trauma Outreach and Prevention An organization that strives for a meaningful world and justice in which every individual enjoys physical, mental and spiritual health. Provides internships and publications in these fields.
Sn: ATOP

Asylum Temporary or permanent stay on its territory, consented by a State to a refugee, stateless person or other persecuted people, with guarantee of their safety and human rights.
Cf. asylum rights, asylum seeker, persecution

Asylum rights Providing asylum is a humanitarian act. According to the 1948 Universal Declaration of Human Rights, it is the right of everyone "to seek asylum and to enjoy in other countries asylum from persecution".
Cf. asylum, asylum seeker, persecution

Asylum seeker A person or community requesting entry into a country for safety, humanitarian or other valid reasons. According to UDHR, it is a right "to seek and to enjoy in other countries asylum from persecution".
Cf. asylum right, refugee, territorial asylum, diplomatic asylum, human rights

Athrepsia Sn: nutritional marasmus

Atmosphere The gaseous and turbulent envelope that englobes the earth.

Atmospheric pollution Presence in the atmosphere of large quantities of gases, solids and radiation produced by the burning of natural and artificial fuels, chemical and other industrial processes and nuclear explosions. To a lesser extent also contamination by accumulation of cosmic dust, surface dust by wind, volcanoes, natural radioactivity, etc.
Cf. acid rain, air pollution, ozone depletion, transboundary pollution

Atmospheric pressure Pressure of the atmosphere that varies according to the latitude and to meteorological conditions. Normal atmospheric pressure is 76 cm of mercury at 0 °C.

Atoll A circular coral reef, generally with one or more low islands, surrounding a central lagoon which may or may not communicate with the ocean.

Atom The smallest particle of matter, in an electrically neutral state, consisting of a positively charged (proton) nucleus, round which revolve negatively charged electrons.
Cf. atomic bomb, nuclear reaction, nuclear reactor

Atomic bomb Atom bomb, or A-bomb, the basic nuclear weapon in which the explosive energy is derived only from fission of the atomic nuclei, liberating energy and radiation. The first atom bombs dropped in 1945 on Hiroshima and Nagasaki, Japan, were of this type.
Sn: atom bomb, A-bomb, fission bomb
Cf. fallout, kiloton, fusion bomb, hydrogen bomb, thermonuclear bomb, nuclear war, uranium, plutonium, mushroom cloud, Hiroshima

Atomic disaster Cf. nuclear disaster

Atomic power plant Sn: nuclear power plant, nuclear reactor

Atomic reactor Sn: nuclear reactor, nuclear power plant, reactor

Attenuation Diminution, reduction, lessening in force of destructiveness or virulence, abatement.
Cf. disaster mitigation

Attac An independent international movement in support of citizens, active in opposing the excesses of free trade and for more equitable alternatives in social, environmental and democratic processes.
Sn: (Full French title:) Association pour une taxation de Transactions financières pour l'Aide aux Citoyens, more generally known under its acronym, attac.
Cf. disaster mitigation

Audit Systematic, documented, independent, periodic examination of an institution to determine whether or to what extent activities comply with the planned and agreed system.

Auschwitz/Buchenwald Two of the many notorious concentration camps set up by the Nazi regime during World War II with an inhuman programme of purifying the nation by exterminating entire populations, where thousands of inmates of all ages and both sexes were herded in appalling conditions, imprisoned without trial or reason, killed in gas chambers or incinerated in death ovens. Among other camps, Dachau and Birkenau also remain notorious. Other dictatorships create other such camps.
Cf. ethnic cleansing, racism, human rights, pogrom, extermination

Autocracy/autocratic Form of anti-democratic government, ruled by a dictator who has absolute self-sustained power and governs and dictates without consideration of the people governed.
Sn: dictatorship
Cf. democracy, plutocracy

Autopsy Post-mortem (after death) examination of a cadaver with the view to determining the cause and mode of death and identity of the body.
Sn: necropsy

Auxiliary health worker A community health assistant or health worker who is experienced but has less than full professional qualifications and needs supervision by qualified personnel.

Auxiliary power unit An electricity generating machine, supplementary to the normal power line, that can be used when the latter fails. Particularly useful in developing countries, first aid tents and situations like refugee camps, where the supply of electricity may be unreliable.

Avaaz A worldwide independent, non-profit, humanitarian information campaign organization that works to ensure that the values, views and actions of the world's people inform and shape global decision-making in a just manner.

Avalanche Sudden slide of a huge mass of snow and ice, usually carrying with it earth, rocks, trees and other debris.

Average In marine insurance, means damage.
Particular average is damage to the goods.
General average: Expenses voluntarily incurred to save a ship and her cargo.

Avian influenza – H5N1 A highly contagious poultry (or other bird) disease due to the influenza virus H5N1 that affected South East Asia in 2003, transmitted to humans with high case fatality.
Cf. International Health Regulations, pandemic

AVPU Emergency acronym for Awake, Verbal response, Part response, Unresponsive. A rapid neurological assessment of a trauma patient when there is no time to do the Glasgow coma scale.
Cf. ABCDE, Glasgow coma scale

B

Bacillary dysentery An acute, severe, intestinal disease due to the Shigella bacillus, type 1, characterized by bloody stools and fever, associated with poor personal hygiene and sanitation in crowded closed communities (ships, refugee camps, jails). Especially frequent in children and often occurring as sudden outbreaks. Transmitted via the faecal-oral route or water-borne through contaminated water supply, either directly through hand contact or indirectly through contaminated food. The term dysentery is often used in a general sense for many non-specific cases of gastroenteritis and diarrhoea.
Cf. enteric diseases, dysentery

Bacillus Calmette-Guérin Better known as BCG, an attenuated and non-virulent vaccine made from bovine *Mycobacterium tuberculosis* used in vaccination against tuberculosis. It is one of the six vaccines used in the WHO Expanded Programme on Immunization.
Sn: BCG
Cf. vaccine, vaccination, EPI, tuberculosis

Backfire In firefighting, a fire started intentionally by the firefighters along the inner edge of the fire-control line with the aim of consuming the fuel in the path of a forest fire, or of changing the direction of the fire's advance

Bactericide Chemical compound that kills bacteria and is used against infections.
Cf. pesticide, virucide

Bag bomb Portable nuclear arm usually stolen or illegal. Also known as nuclear bag, Bombe valise.

Ballistic missile A pilotless rocket-propelled projectile boosted into space and whose thrust can be terminated at a chosen time, after which its re-entry vehicle returns it to the earth's atmosphere. BM with a range of over 5,500 km is called intercontinental missile (e.g. ICBM) and under 500 km, a strategic missile.
Cf. antiballistic missile, ABM Treaty, arms race, START

Barcelona Declaration Declaration made in 1995, emphasizing the role of diverse cultures in health, promotes dialogue between civilizations and traditions and encourages regional scientific and technological exchanges as essential factors in improving understanding between people and health.

Barefoot doctor In a developing country, a rural-level primary healthcare provider, usually chosen and culturally accepted by the community he or she lives in. System introduced in China during the Cultural Revolution.
Cf. barehead doctor

Barehead doctor In the rural areas of Thailand, Buddhist monks are trained to deliver simple, primary health care at low cost and according to the country's traditions.
Cf. barefoot doctor

Barrier Geography: In the polar regions, the mass of ice formed by the freezing of sea water.
Cf. ice pack, pack ice

Firefighting: Any obstruction to the spread of fire, usually a strip of land free from any combustible material. Cf. firebreak

Bartonellosis An infectious disease endemic in the high valleys of the Andes, transmitted at night by the bite of insects.

Sn: Oroya fever, verruga peruana

Basal metabolic rate The minimal rate of energy production, representing the energy requirements of the body at rest. A measure of the function of the thyroid gland, which is very susceptible to radiation uptake.

Sn: BMR

Cf. calorie, goitre, Lugol's iodine

Basel Accords Beginning in 1974 and reinforced in 2010, a series of financial negotiations establishing international guidelines and rules on security of the world banking system to maintain sufficient shares and capital to cushion against eventual disastrous economic crises, like the one in 2008.

Basel Convention International instrument operated by the United Nations Environment Programme to reduce transboundary movements of hazardous wastes, to minimize such material, to control their moves and incidents and to assist in environmental management in developing countries.

Cf. chemical accident, environmental pollution, hazardous material, International Programme on Chemical Safety

Basic health care The provision of the minimal, simplified essential health requirements in a low-income country, based on essential vaccination, essential medicaments and simple perinatal care, not necessarily integrated within the country's organized basic health

services and socioeconomic needs. It should be distinguished from Primary Health Care.

Cf. Primary Health Care, essential surgery

Basic life support/BLS An advanced form of non-invasive first aid to a person who is critically ill or has a severe injury in order to ensure the ABC of survival, i.e. Airway clearance, Breathing maintained and Circulation assured. These are the first elements of cardiopulmonary resuscitation – Safar.

Sn: BLS

Cf. ABC, advanced life support, cardiopulmonary resuscitation, survival chain

Basic societal functions In any given society, the significant functions that may affect – or be affected by – actions and circumstances that may result in disorder, disaster, injustice or loss of human rights. Inter alia, these may include a country's legal structure, governance, security, education, economy, health and sanitation systems, water and shelter, public works, food, energy and communications, transport, distribution and level of social participation.

BCG Sn: Bacillus Calmette-Guérin

Beaufort scale Numerical scale from 0 to 12, indicating wind force.

0 calm, 1 light air, 2 light breeze, 3 gentle breeze, 4 moderate breeze, 5 fresh breeze, 6 strong breeze, 7 strong wind, 8 gale, 9 strong gale, 10 storm, 11 violent storm, 12 hurricane.

Cf. Douglas scale, gale, hurricane, storm, wind, Saffir-Simpson scale

Beijing Declaration, 1995 Beijing Declaration and Platform for Action. The 4th World Conference on Women, UNESCO, set positive gender standards and obligations in favour of women.

Beneficiary Person, group or country that receives the aid or services of others.
Sn: donee
Cf. aid, international assistance

Beriberi A severe nutritional deficiency of vitamin B_1 mainly seen in areas where the basic diet is polished rice (South East Asia). It is characterized by neuritis, oedema, muscular atrophy and cardiac failure.
Sn: vitamin B_1 deficiency
Cf. nutritional deficiency

Bermuda triangle Cf. intertropical convergence zone

Bhopal disaster Major technological/industrial disaster that took place in the town of Bhopal, India, on 3 December 1984, when large quantities of highly toxic methyl isocyanate escaped from a damaged chemical factory, causing over 2,000 deaths and thousands others disabled, in respiratory distress and blind. The worst chemical disaster to date. Compensations are still pending.
Cf. man-made disaster, technological disaster, Chernobyl, Seveso

Bifurcated needle A special two-pronged needle used in vaccination to deliver equal doses of vaccine. Was particularly used in global smallpox vaccination.

Big One, The A hypothetical devastating earthquake of 8.3 Richter over the San Andreas Fault in California predicted to have 50% probability of striking the San Francisco Bay area within the coming quarter century.
Cf. fault, sliding fault, Richter scale

Bilateral cooperation Technical cooperation or assistance given by a donor country to a recipient country, through direct agreement between the two governments, without UN or other intermediary.

Cf. international assistance, technical assistance

Bilateralism In international or intergovernmental relations, the conduct of doing business or negotiations between two States or organizations, in respectful consideration of the positions of both.
Cf. multilateralism, unilateralism

Bilharzia Sn: schistosomiasis

Bill and Melinda Gates Foundation Richly endowed foundation with particular action against the major communicable and socially disruptive diseases, in close collaboration with WHO and the World Bank, through imaginative funding systems.
Sn: Gates Foundation
Cf. GAVI, Global fund, World Bank

Binary weapon A chemical arm which is not lethal until two chemical compounds are mixed in the detonation moment.
Cf. chemical war

Bio From the Greek *bios*, life; prefix denoting life, living, organic life. Example: biology

Bioburden Bacteriological contamination complicating a wound or a patient's condition.

Biodiversity The global sum total of all the varieties of living genes, organisms, species and ecosystems on earth. Its preservation is absolutely essential to human well-being and the earth's health, yet it is under constant threat.

Bioethics A term made of the Greek words bios (life) and ethos (ethics). In health care and life sciences, the systematic study and consideration of human conduct in relation to principles and moral values, with attention to the person and the person's humanity.

Biogeography The science that deals with the causes, modifications and interactions of geographical distribution of living organisms on earth.

Biological agents classification Biological agents/weapons are usually classified (a) according to their taxonomy: fungi bacteria and viruses; (b) according to their infectivity, virulence, lethality, pathogenicity, incubation period; (c) according to their contagiousness and mechanism of transmission; and (d) according to their stability or capacity of survival.
Cf. chemical agents classification, chemical weapons, biological warfare

Biological and chemical weapons The two are usually considered together.
Cf. chemical and biological weapons, biological weapons, chemical weapons

Biological disaster Disaster caused by a large-scale exposure of the biomass or living organisms to toxic substances, germs or radiation.
Cf. biomass, biological warfare, environ-mental disaster, man-made disaster, technological disaster, toxicological disaster

Biological equilibrium Condition in which the interactions between the different animal and vegetable species is such that the structure and function of an ecosystem remain fairly constant.
Man is the main element in the modifications of this equilibrium.
Cf. ecosystem, biodiversity

Biological hazard A source of potential damage of varying degrees caused by living organisms, including pathogenic microorganisms, saprophytes, vaccines and other biological substances that may cause injury, loss of life, social disruption, economic disturbance and environmental degradation.
Cf. biological disaster, hazard

Biological warfare The intentional spread of disease in warfare through the dispersal of infective bacteria, rickettsiae, viruses, toxins or other biological weapons which cause diseases such as anthrax, plague, typhoid, brucellosis.
There is a UN Convention against biological weapons. Biological and chemical weapons are considered together (CBW) as weapons of mass destruction.
Sn: bacteriological warfare, biological weapon, BW
Cf. bioterrorism, chemical warfare, nuclear war, toxin, CBW

Biological weapons Weapons that achieve their intended target effects through the infectivity of disease-causing microorganisms and other replicative entities, including viruses, infectious nucleic acids, prions – WHO.
The Biological Weapons Convention requires states parties "never in any circumstances to develop, produce, stockpile or otherwise acquire or retain (1) microbial or other biological agents or toxins … and (2) weapons equipment or means of delivery designed to use such agents or toxins for hostile purposes or in armed conflict" – BWC.
Cf. biological warfare, Biological Weapons Convention, chemical weapons, CBW

Biological Weapons Convention/CBW United Nations Convention on the Prohibition of the Development, Production and Stockpiling of Bacteriological (Biological) and Toxic Weapons and their Destruction, signed in 1972.
Cf. biological warfare, biological weapons, chemical warfare, man-conceived disaster, bioterrorism, terrorism, CBW, weapons of mass destruction

Biomass The total quantity of the living matter of organisms present in a given environment at a given time.
It is expressed in volume, in mass (dry weight, fresh weight, decalcified or not), in carbon, in calories per unit of volume or of surface.
Sn: standing crop

Biosphere The biotic environment of the earth where life can be maintained and supported by ecosystems, including the hydrosphere, the lower part of the atmosphere, the upper part of the ionosphere and, by extension, of the totality of living matter on earth.
Cf. ecosystem

Bioterrorism Planning, threatening, using or spreading contagious disease organisms or toxin, e.g. botulism, anthrax, viruses, debilitating war gases, as a terrorist tool or weapon.
Cf. terrorism, biological warfare, chemical warfare, man-conceived disaster, CBW

Birth rate Ratio between the number of births during a given period and the total size of the population.
Cf. death rate

bit Acronym for BInary digiT. The smallest unit of information with which a digital computer works

Black tide Cf. oil slick

Bleaching powder Calcium hypochlorite
Cf. chlorine

BLEVE Acronymic name for boiling liquid expanded vapour explosion.
The sudden rupture of a closed vessel system containing liquefied petroleum gas (LPG) flammable under intense pressure due to flame impingement, creating a blast wave, missile projectile damage and immediate ignition of the expanding fuel-air mixture leading to a disastrous fireball. Examples: Los Alfaques in Spain, Mexico City.
Cf. fire, fire hazard

Blizzard Violent and very cold wind laden with snow, at least some part of which has been raised from snow-covered ground.
Cf. wind, winter blizzard

Blood bank A special section or part of a laboratory, usually in a hospital, which has the scientific facilities to receive and store human blood and blood components from a blood centre – while often it may itself be the blood centre. It performs blood compatibility testing and provides blood and blood products to hospitals and transfusion centres. It may be called the transfusion laboratory.

Blood diamonds The valuable and expensive stone, the diamond, that plays an important role in the economy and development of its producing countries is also used for illegal and unethical purposes such as purchasing arms, funding conflicts, supplying armies, providing influence, fomenting rebellions or financing dictatorships, thus being referred to as blood diamonds or conflict diamonds. The Kimberley Process Certification Scheme was set up in 2003 by governments and the diamond industry to stop the illegal trade in rough diamonds that help buy influence or pay rebel groups, civil wars and totalitarian régimes, mainly in Africa.
The term extends also to other precious metals and expensive products, such as blood copper or blood rubber.
Sn: conflict diamonds

Blood products Any therapeutic substance derived from human blood, including whole blood, plasma, plasma-derived products and labile blood components, used for medical purposes.

Boat people People who due to persecution, insecurity, poverty or any other reason flee a country by boat and seek security or asylum in another country. They are usually subjected to much suffering, disease, danger on the high seas, administrative complications or refusal to land.

Cf. displaced persons, refugee, high seas

Body mass index/BMI A measure of weight in relation to height. Calculated as weight in kg, divided by the square of height in metres. A BMI of less than 25 is considered normal, 25–30 is overweight, greater than 30 is obesity. Used in nutritional assessment.

Cf. obesity

Body surface area/BSA Assessment of the burnt surface area of the body in a thermal injury. BSA is usually expressed in sections of 9% (the rule of 9) of the body area burnt. Less frequently, it is also expressed mathematically:

$$\sqrt{\frac{BSA\left(m^2\right) = Ht\left(cm\right) \times Wt\left(kg\right)}{3600}}$$

Cf. burn, burn extent, rule of 9, burn degrees, burn disaster

Booby trap A military or a terrorist improvised device designed to explode on being manipulated, e.g. when a person opens a door, starts up a car or picks up a parcel.

Cf. terrorism, landmines

Botulism Cf. food poisoning

Bovine spongiform encephalopathy/ BSE Cf. mad cow disease, Creutzfeldt-Jakob disease

Bradford disaster scale To facilitate comparison of one disaster with another, the BDS defines magnitudes by taking the logarithm (base 100) of the number of fatalities.

Supplementary to magnitude, a classification system can be introduced – Keller.

Fatalities	Disaster	Deaths	Class	Magnitude
0–10			0	0
$10–10^2$	Bangkok	166	1	1.73
$10^2–10^3$	Zeebrugge	187	2	2.27
$10^3–10^4$	Bhopal	2,000	3	3.30
$10^4–10^5$	Armenia	24,000	4	44.38
$10^5–10^6$			5	

Cf. disaster severity scales

Brain death A traumatic condition in which electroencephalography reveals no cortical brain activity. A vegetative state in which the heart may continue beating.

Breeder reactor A nuclear reactor facility which produces more fissile nuclei than it consumes.

Briand-Kellogg Pact League of Nations Pact of 1928 that condemns the "recourse" to war for the "settlement" of international disputes as an instrument of national politics in international relations.

Cf. crime of aggression

Brock Chisholm Memorial Trust Scientific and humanitarian institution established in 1984 at WHO by Grace B. Chisholm and S. William Gunn to honour the legacy of Dr. George Brock Chisholm of Canada, first Director-General of the World Health Organization, and to perpetuate his ideals and vision of humanism, health, international understanding and peace. Subsequently, the Trust has been incorporated as the International Association for Humanitarian Medicine Brock Chisholm (IAHM).

Cf. International Association for Humanitarian Medicine, humanitarian medicine

Brucellosis A febrile zoonotic disease caused by eating unpasteurized milk or dairy products from infected animals.
Sn: Malta fever, Mediterranean fever, zoonosis

Buffering The capacity of a society or community to protect itself from the damaging effects of a disaster, or to prepare itself to minimize the effects of an expected disaster. Cf. Attenuation.
In geopolitics, a smaller zone or country between two larger belligerent countries, diminishing the chances of hostilities.

Building code(s) A series of governmental and professional regulations setting technical and functional standards for the built environment, especially concerning materials, structure, design, aesthetics, safety, salubrity and social welfare.
Cf. built environment, retrofitting

Built environment Within the context of mainly exploitable land, any and all physical structures built by man, including houses, factories, roads, electric lines, satellite antennas, underground wires, communication tunnels, sewers, ports, dams, bridges, farmhouses or sheds, airports, railways, schools, recreation grounds, municipal structures, etc., as distinct from the natural environment.
Cf. building codes

Bulghur Boiled, dried and crushed wheat with outside bran removed, used for food. Total cooked whole wheat.
Cf. conventional food

Burden of disease In the assessment of health levels or a health system, an indicator that quantifies losses of healthy life from disease and injury.

Double burden represents a large number of non-communicable diseases coinciding with large numbers of communicable diseases, malnutrition and maternal mortality.
Cf. disability-adjusted life expectancy, disease surveillance, ten-ninety disequilibrium

Burn Tissue damage of varying degrees caused by the heat produced from a thermal agent. Burns are classified according to the extent of body surface involved, according to the depth of tissue damage, or according to the cause, e.g. flame, steam, electric, chemical, lightning, nuclear radiation
Cf. chemical burn, electrical burn, burn degree, burn extent, Euro-Mediterranean Council for Burns and Fire Disasters, thermal agent disaster

Burn, chemical Cf. chemical burn

Burn classification Cf. burn

Burn, degrees On a burnt patient, three degrees of burns are distinguished, according to the depth of the burnt area, important in the healing process and treatment. First degree: damage limited to the outer superficial layer of the epidermis, with redness and pain, e.g. sunburn; 2nd: the burn extends through the epidermis down to dermis, but not entirely compromising the regeneration process; 3rd: full-thickness burn, killing the skin. These degrees concern the depth and not the extent of the area burnt.
Cf. burn, burn rule of 9

Burn disaster The overall effect on living persons or animals, caused by massive burn action from a known thermal agent, characterized by a large number of immediate deaths and burnt patients and a high rate of

secondary   mortality   and
disability – Masellis.
Cf. thermal agent disaster, burn, burn
centre.

Burn extent – Rule of 9 In a burned
person, the body's surface area
(BSA) that is burnt has great importance in the outcome of the injury
and treatment. For practical calculations, the body is divided into areas,
each representing 9% of its surface.
Thus, the head represents 9%, an
arm 9%, a leg 18%, the back 18%,
etc. (This assessment – of surface –
is different from the degree of
burn.)
Cf. burn, burn degree, body surface
area,   thermal   injury,   Euro-
Mediterranean Council for Burns and
Fire Disasters

Burns Centre Particular unit and facilities in a hospital for the specialized
care for all aspects of severely burned
patients, including surgical, reconstructive, nursing, medico-social, rehabilitative and other ancillary facilities
for a large number of patients. It also
promotes burns prevention in the community and collaborates closely with
the authorities in firefighting and preparedness programmes.
Cf. emergency   medical   services,
fires

Burn out A state of physical and psychological exhaustion that a person
presents in response to the heavy
stress and difficulties of unrelenting
performance expended or demanded
in the individual's occupation. This is
not   uncommon   among   disaster
responders who often work under
most unfavourable and strenuous
conditions.

Buruli ulcer A destructive skin infection   caused   by   *Mycobacterium*

ulcerans that belongs to the same
family of organisms that cause leprosy
and tuberculosis. A neglected tropical
disease.
Cf. neglected tropical diseases

C

Caesium A naturally occurring isotope
in the earth's crust. Atomic number
55, symbol Cs. Cesium-137 is a
product of atomic fission of uranium
and an important component of radioactive fallout.
Cf. uranium, plutonium, fallout

Calcium   hypochlorite Bleaching
powder, chlorine.
Cf. chlorine

Camp Lodgings in tents or temporary
quarters. Camps are erected for (i)
refugees, (ii) displaced persons in
time of peace, (iii) persons displaced
in time of conflict. (The HCR prefers
not to use the term camps for refugees.) Prohibited camps are concentration   camps,   forced   grouping,
forced labour camps, extermination
camps.

Canadair Originally the commercial
brand name of a firefighting air
tanker, now used generically for any
water discharging aircraft.

**Canadian International Development
Authority** Commonly referred to as
CIDA,   important   governmental
department devoted to the study,
development of products, institutions, progress and governance in
poorer States and sustainable growth
in developing countries; includes
disaster prevention and emergency
aid. (Not to be confused with SIDA.)

Cancerogenic That causes cancer, neo-
plastic disease or malignant growth.
Sn: carcinogenic

Cancun Agreements Follow-up to the Kyoto Protocol, establishing clear and verifiable obligations on States concerning high carbon dioxide emissions and their effects on climate and developing countries.
Cf. Kyoto protocol, global warming, carbon dioxide, climate change

Capacity building Methods and ends of increasing the aggregate ability of a person, community or nation in individual skills, institutional capacity, organizational structures, economic means, governmental leadership, education, human resources, citizen participation and resilience with the view to strengthening society in face of risks, disasters and other challenges.
Cf. disaster preparedness, resilience

Cape Town Declaration Beginning in 1999, the UN started building bridges to the private sector through the Global Compact. The 2007 Cape Town Declaration strengthened this process by innovative UN partnerships with NGOs and the private sector with commitment to corporate social responsibility and a stronger engagement in the Millennium Development Goals.
Cf. Global compact, Millennium Development Goals

Carbon capture Carbon capture and storage (CCS) is a new technology to tackle the world's increasing rate of carbon dioxide emissions, with resulting atmospheric and climate change.

Carbon dioxide – CO$_2$ A colourless gas produced by complete combustion of carbon, by thermal decomposition and during fermentation. It is essential to metabolism – exhaled by animals and absorbed by plants. Important role in climate change.

Major component of industrial and automobile emissions.
Cf. glasshouse effect, Kyoto protocol, Cancun agreements, global warming, climate change

Carbon monoxide – CO Odourless poisonous gas, a product of incomplete combustion. May be fatal if formed under conditions of limited supply of air, as in a closed room.

Carcinogenic Chemical, viral, radioactive or other agent that can induce cancer or malignant disease in man or in other organisms.
Sn: cancerogenic

Cardiac arrest The stopping of blood circulation with disappearance of blood pressure and cessation of heart function. Commonly called heart attack.
Cf. first aid, basic life support

Cardiopulmonary-cerebral resuscitation In a severely ill or seriously injured person, providing the essential life needs for survival through manoeuvres that ensure emergency oxygenation, restoration of spontaneous blood circulation and cerebral resuscitation.
Sn: CPR
Cf. basic life support

Cardiopulmonary resuscitation The technique and manoeuvres applied to a severely injured patient in order to ensure the basic functions of the heart and lungs and to maintain such vital support until the end of the critical period.
Sn: emergency intensive care, CPR, critical care
Cf. emergency critical services, first aid, rescue

Caritas Internationalis Confederation of many national Catholic charity organizations to provide relief, social aid and justice in the world. Member of the Vatican Pontifical Council Cor Unum.

Cf. humanitarian, international assistance

Carrier A person or animal who harbours an infection without knowing it and without clinical signs of disease and who serves as a potential source of involuntary transmission to other persons. A healthy carrier may be in an incubation period or may be completely ignorant of any disease, while the convalescent carrier is himself cured but may transmit the disease.

Cf. incubation period, source of infection, quarantine

Cartagena Protocol on Biodiversity International treaty on Biodiversity (2000), the first such legally binding environmental instrument. It seeks to protect biological diversity from potential risks of genetically modified organisms (GMO), regulating their transboundary movements and maintaining biosafety centres.

Cf. biodiversity, genetically modified organisms

Cartel Politics: An understanding (usually secret) between political bodies, trade unions and other similar organizations with the view to more effective concerted action.

Economics: A secret understanding or antisocial agreement (often criminal) between commercial or industrial bodies to ensure monopoly, domination of the market prices and high profits.

Cf. Palermo protocol, mafia

Carter Center A special section of the Jimmy Carter Foundation Presidential Library devoted to the advancement of human rights and humanitarian causes, alleviation of suffering, equity in governance and conflict resolution.

Case fatality rate The calculation of the number of patients dying from a specific disease, divided by the number of individuals developing that disease. It is usually expressed per 1,000 affected persons

Cassava The root of two plants of the spurge or manioc family (bitter and sweet cassava), the flour of which is used for bread and is an important source of food starch in many countries.

Sn: manioc

Cf. staple food

Casualty Any victim of any emergency health situation, without specifying the gravity or nature of the emergency. May concern a sharp abdominal pain, a cut, burn, heart attack, fracture, fall, poisoning, drowning, fainting, shock, head injury or any other acute episode, minor, serious or lethal that has called for some attention and necessary care. Often in disaster statistics, the term is erroneously used for the seriously injured and dead.

In the UK, the Casualty Department is the general Emergency Department of a hospital.

Cf. accident, mass casualty situation, hospital capacity

Cataclysmic An exaggerated term from the Greek for the Biblical deluge. Describes a very severe, extensive disaster. It has no practical value and should not be used.

Cf. catastrophic, Hiroshima, Bhopal, Chernobyl

Catastrophe Sn: disaster

Catastrophe theory A mathematical and philosophical theory that tries to explain and define transitional discontinuity according to which a disaster represents a sudden, brutal break and change in the forces present in natural, physical, social or psychological phenomena – Thom.
Cf. chaos theory

Catastrophic Catastrophe and disaster are synonymous. The adjectival form "catastrophic" is sometimes used to describe a very extensive disaster. Such exaggerated, figurative terms, including "cataclysmic", have no practical value and are not recommended.
The term "catastrophic fires", however, denotes the simultaneous coalescence of multiple fires or firestorm (Cf)

Catastrophic fire General term for the simultaneous coalescing of multiple fires, or firestorm.

Catastrophic health spending A situation "when the proportion of people spends out-of-pocket more than 40% of their incomes for health after deducting expenses for food each year" – WHO.
The situation hits particularly the poorer people and poor families with a disabled member.

Catchment area Sn: catchment basin, river basin

Catchment basin Sn: river basin

Caveat In Latin: "Let him or her beware" or "be careful". A warning notice to the reader to be aware of something possibly misleading, or possible confusion between two terms. Particularly important in international texts of varying languages.

Central depression Vast meteorological and barometric depression, usually stationary or semistatic, within which smaller depressions circulate.
Cf. depression

Centre Europe-Tiers Monde/Europe-Third World Centre (CETIM)
The Europe-Third World Centre is an NGO dedicated to the defence and promotion of all human rights, on the principle that these rights are inseparable and indivisible. Publishes useful guides in these fields at University of Lausanne.
Cf. third world, human rights, development

Centre for International Health and Cooperation/CIHC A think-and-action group at Fordham University based on the precept that health and other humanitarian endeavours may sometimes provide the only common ground for initiating dialogue, understanding and cooperation among people and nations at war or in conflict. The Centre directs the International Diploma in Humanitarian Assistance (IDHA).

Centre for Research on the Epidemiology of Disasters A pioneering facility at the School of Public Health, Catholic University of Louvain, Belgium, for research, study and training in the epidemiology and medical aspects of disasters. A WHO Collaborating Centre.
Sn: CRED
Cf. disaster medicine, epidemiology

Center for the Study of Bioterrorism and Emerging Infections Major centre at Saint Louis University, USA, on all aspects of military and bacteriological epidemiology of bioterrorist threats and biodefence.
Cf. bioterrorism, biological weapons, anthrax

Cerebral haemorrhage Bleeding into the brain. A serious condition that can be due to circulatory disease, or to skull injury, as in entrapment in an earthquake.

Cerebrospinal meningitis Very serious, highly contagious neurological infection attacking the envelope (meninges) of the brain and of the spine. Can attain epidemic proportions.
Cf. encephalitis

Chagas disease A chronic infection caused by trypanosomes, characterized by irregular fever, swelling of lymph glands, oedema, skin eruptions and, in advanced stages, by apathy, convulsions and coma. It may appear in acute form in children. Predominant in South America and Africa, spreads through blood-sucking flies, infected blood transfusion, organ transplantation. A neglected tropical disease.
Sn: sleeping sickness, American trypanosomiasis

Chaos theory A mathematical theory and technique applied to non-linear dynamics to ascertain the changing structure or pattern that underlies certain apparently random observations, as in wind, fire, waves, hazardous chemical propagation or even human behaviour.
Cf. catastrophe theory

Charity Altruistic action in a variety of fields and ways, by an individual or organization, to help, relieve, soothe and advance a cause, a public need, persons or communities in distress.
Cf. altruism, voluntary organization

Chartering In transport and shipping, the contract or hire of a ship or airplane or of part of the vessel.
Sn: charter party, freighting

Charter party Sn: chartering

Chatham House Rules An undertaking by participants in a conference or discussion proceedings that one can report on what was said at the meeting but cannot give the name or affiliation of the person who said it. This is based on the core principle that governs confidentiality of the source of information.

Chauvinism Excessive, aggressive patriotism; the belief that one's country is the best in everything and cannot be criticized.

Chemical accident Accidental release outside its accepted confines that may occur during research, production, transportation or handling of toxic or other hazardous chemical substances, dangerous to human health and/or the environment in the short or long term. Also referred to as chemical incident. Such events include fires, explosions, leakages or terrorism.
Cf. corrosion burn, environmental pollution, hazmat, International Programme on Chemical Safety

Chemical agents classification Classification of harmful chemicals may take several paths: (a) according to the degree of effect, e.g. harassing, lethal or incapacitating; (b) according to the route of entry, e.g. respiratory agents, cutaneous agents; (c) according to the duration of the hazard, e.g. persistent agents, non-persistent, temporary.
Cf. chemical agents/weapons, biological agents classification

Chemical agents/weapons Chemical agents are weapons that are effective because of their toxicity, i.e. their chemical action on life processes

capable of causing death, temporary incapacitation or permanent harm. Some toxic chemicals such as phosgene, hydrogen cyanide and tear gas may be used for both civil and peaceful, as well as for hostile purposes. In the latter case, they too are chemical weapons – WHO.
Cf. chemical weapons, biological weapons, Chemical Weapons Convention, riot-control gases

Chemical and biological weapons The two are usually studied together, with considerations of lethal effects, incapacitating effects, harassing effects. (Cf. these terms.)

Chemical burn Destruction of human tissue due to the action of chemical agents. Also called corrosion burn. For exposure to corrosive substances with skin damage, classification can be made according to the principles applying to thermal burn injuries, as follows (IPCS): Group 1, life threatening injury: dermal and full-thickness injuries exceeding 50% of body surface area; Group 2a, severe injury: full-thickness injuries of 10–50% or dermal injuries of 20–50% BSA; Group 2b, moderate injury: full-thickness injuries of 2–10% or dermal injuries of 10–20% BSA; Group 3, mild injury: full-thickness injuries 2% BSA, or dermal injuries less than 10% BSA or epidermal injuries.
Cf. body surface area, burn disaster, chemical accident, thermal injury, corrosion, International Programme on Chemical Safety

Chemical hazard A chemical product that, on exposure, may cause health problems to persons or communities.

Chemical warfare War in which harmful chemical substances are used with the intention to kill, injure, or otherwise incapacitate humans or to destroy the environment and national economies. A weapon of mass destruction.
The many chemical weapons are grouped in seven main categories in terms of their toxic properties: nerve agents (lethal), cyanide (lethal), tissue damaging vesicants (mustards, lewisites, halogenated oximes), psychotomimetics, riot control agents (incapacitating) and defoliants. Chemical weapons are internationally outlawed by the 1925 Geneva Protocol.
Sn: chemical weapon, CW
Cf. Chemical Weapons Convention, Geneva Conventions, GLAWARS, International Humanitarian Law, biological warfare, defoliant, agent orange, weapons of mass destruction, WMD

Chemical weapons According to the Chemical Weapons Convention, "chemical weapons" means the following together or separately: (a) toxic chemicals and their precursors... (b) munitions and devices specifically designed to cause death or other harm through their toxic properties...and (c) any equipment specifically designed for use directly in connection with the employment of munitions and devices specified above – CWC.
Cf. toxic chemical, chemical agents, biological weapons, bioterrorism, weapon of mass destruction

Chemical Weapons Convention/ CWC More exactly the Convention on the Prohibition of Chemical

Weapons (CWC) that entered into force in 1997 defines "chemical weapons" and "toxic chemicals" that are or may be used as weapons, sets measures of prohibition, establishes elaborate provisions on verification and also describes a list of chemicals not prohibited under the Convention. Cf. chemical weapons, toxic chemicals, chemical warfare

Chemoprophylaxis The administration of chemotherapeutic medicaments to a susceptible or contaminated person or germ carrier for the purpose of preventing the development of a clinical infection in him.

Chernobyl A town in Ukraine, site of a nuclear reactor that, during mechanical inspection, exploded and burned on 26 April 1986, causing radioactive contamination locally and in distant countries, with deaths, birth anomalies and agricultural and environmental damage extending far afield and over many years, still continuing. The whole reactor (No. 4) has been permanently covered under a heavy concrete sarcophagus and put definitively out of action. However, over time, this having proved insufficient, an all-steel sarcophagus is to be installed. The most serious nuclear disaster to this date, highest (level 7) on the INES scale. It resulted also in IAEA's extensive revision, strengthening and continuous supervision of all nuclear facilities.
Cf. Three Mile Island, Sellafield, Windscale, Fukushima, reactor, man-made disaster, sarcophagus, concrete encasement, International Nuclear Event Scale, International Atomic Energy Agency

Chikungunya fever A viral fever transmitted by the mosquito *Aedes albopictus*.

Presents with headaches, joint pains, diarrhoea and vomiting with dehydration. Infrequent but sudden epidemics, e.g. La Réunion, 2006.

Child Every person under the age of 18 years (unless under national law applicable to the child, majority is attained earlier) – Rights of the Child, 1989.
Every human being under the age of 18. The age limit, below which it should not be permitted to deprive a child of his or her liberty, should be determined by law – UN.
Sn: minor, juvenile
Cf. child abuse, child protection, child soldier, child prostitution, human rights, UN Declaration of the Rights of the Child

Child abuse An action or situation in which a child's development is threatened or stunted due to systematically bad treatment, neglect, emotional harassment, sexual or other physical assaults, by a perpetrator who is a caretaker or family member.
Cf. child, child protection, child neglect, child soldier, UN Declaration on the Rights of the Child

Child deaths tragedy Nearly 11 million children under 5 die every year, mostly from diseases that are preventable.

Child neglect The child has the right to food, housing, clothing, medical care and adequate leisure to grow normally. Not providing these facilities constitutes neglect, punishable by law. The rights are applicable even under difficult circumstances, such as in a disaster situation.
Cf. child, UN Declaration on the Rights of the Child, Save the Children

Child prostitution The use of a child in sexual activities for remuneration or any other form of consideration – UN.

Child protection The necessary surveillance, care, protection and comfort provided to children who are at risk of abuse, neglect, army enlistment, sexual traffic or abandonment, or who have already suffered from such maltreatment.
Cf. child, child abuse, Universal Declaration of Human Rights

Child soldiers Children and minor age boys are being increasingly recruited, encouraged or forced into joining armed forces in several belligerent countries, especially in revolutionary armies, insurgent troops or illegal fighting groups, with extremely harmful effects on the children concerned and on their families. This is against all international law and the rights of the child and must be denounced.

Chlorine Chemically calcium hypochlorite, also called bleaching powder, a generally available chemical substance used for disinfection of water and waste products. Differently prepared solutions or powders are used for water chlorination (water purification, using 0.7 mg/l) and for disinfection of solids, such as powdering the latrines in a refugee community. Its excessive use in industry can cause severe environmental pollution.
Sn: bleaching powder, calcium hypochlorite
Cf. environment, hygiene, environmental pollution

Chlorofluorocarbons (CFC) A group of chemical compounds used in industry and in the household, mainly as the propelling agent in hairsprays, shaving foam, etc. Their excessive and universal use is believed to be one of the causes of ozone depletion, with resulting environmental damage.

Cf. ozone depletion, greenhouse effect

Chloroquine A classical quinine derivative that has been successful against malaria, but which has induced chloroquine resistance, with reduced effect.
Cf. mefloquine, quinine, malaria

Cholera A severe, acute infection of the intestines, characterized by profuse watery diarrhoea, vomiting, dehydration, muscle cramps and collapse. It is spread by the ingestion of food and water contaminated by the faeces of infected (symptomatic or asymptomatic) persons.
Several diarrhoeal diseases are diagnosed as cholera, but the latter is caused by the *Vibrio cholerae*. It is subject to international quarantine regulations.
Cf. cholera vaccine, diarrhoeal diseases, quarantine

Cholera vaccine A vaccine administered against cholera. It is of limited value and, in disaster situations, sanitary measures rather than vaccination suffice.

Chromosome The complex essential structure of the living cell nucleus containing deoxyribonucleic acid (DNA) molecules. Chromosome aberration is any mutation of a chromosome due to toxic or radiation accidents that may result in harmful changes to the organism. The Y-chromosome designates the male sex, while the X-chromosome is paired in both male and female sexes.
Cf. genetic aberration, radioactive contamination, DNA

Ciguatera Human illness that often appears after tsunamis, caused by the absorption of toxins or marine animals, especially fish and crustaceans, characterized by gastrointestinal disturbance, nausea, vomiting and diarrhoea.

It also seemed to appear following coral destruction from nuclear bomb testing in the Pacific Ocean.
Cf. diarrhoeal diseases, toxin, tsunami

Circulatory failure An adverse situation in a person when the cardiovascular system cannot provide sufficient oxygen and nutrients to the body's vital organs and remove the used metabolites.
Cf. cardiac arrest, ABC

Circumcision Male: Removal of the penile foreskin. May be for traditional, religious or medical reasons. Female: Removal of the clitoris and labia in different forms. All are female genital mutilation.
Cf. female genital mutilation

Civil defence The system of measures, usually run by a governmental agency, to protect the civilian population in wartime and to prevent and mitigate the consequences of major emergencies in peacetime. The wider term civil protection is now preferred.
Cf. civil protection, International Civil Defence Organization

Civil disturbance Hostile confrontation among the population, for various reasons; conflict within the social order, with protests and unruly actions on the public domain; may degenerate into riots and need the intervention of the forces of order. May follow a tense disaster situation or may be the fair expression of justice against oppression.

Civil liberties The fundamental legal rights of all citizens to think, decide and act on their own, without state interference and without curtailing the rights of other citizens.
Cf. civil rights, Universal Declaration of Human Rights

Civil protection The organized actions of planning, training, preparedness and response to all emergencies at the local and national levels, with the view to protecting the civilian population in case of natural catastrophe, man-made disaster or war. As a wider, all-hazards approach, the term is now preferred to and covers civil defence.
Cf. civil defence, International Civil Defence Organization

Civil rights According to international laws, it is the right of everyone, without distinction of race, colour, nationality or ethnic origin, to enjoy civil equality before the law, notably the following rights: (a) the right to equal treatment before the tribunal and justice; (b) the right to security and protection; (c) political rights; (d) other civil rights, in particular (i) freedom of movement and residence in one's State, (ii) to leave the country and return, (iii) nationality, (iv) marriage and choice of spouse, (v) own property, (vi) to inherit, (vii) freedom of thought, conscience and religion, (viii) opinion and expression, (ix) peaceful assembly and association; (e) economic, social and cultural rights, in particular (i) choice of work and employment, (ii) form and join trade unions, (iii) housing, (iv) public health, medical care, social security and social services, (v) education and training, (vi) equal participation in cultural activities; (f) the right of access to any place or service for the general public.
Cf. human rights

Civil society The aggregate of a very wide gamut of social and public organizations and structures, of any size or nature, within a society, that respond to a community's or citizens' multifaceted needs and civil expectations, but exclude force, governmental, judiciary, military, police or ecclesiastic elements.

Civil war A much used but ill-clarified term, not defined in the Geneva Conventions. It refers to a war between organized armed insurgent opposition groups and the regular armed forces within the same nation or State. A recent definition is 'non-international armed conflict'.
Cf. war, armed conflict, guerilla, Geneva Conventions

Class of fire Fires can be classified according to size, according to the kind of fuel, whether natural or man-made, domestic or industrial, etc. Four classes are distinguished according to the kind of fuel and the resulting type of extinguishing, as follows:
Class A: Fires started from common combustibles, such as paper, wood, which require cooling, such as with water, retardants, etc.
Class B: Fires involving combustibles or inflammable liquid or gases, which require air exclusion for extinction.
Class C: Fires caused by electricity.
Class D: Fires due to some combustible metal, such as sodium, potassium, which are extinguishable by heat absorption.

Classification of chemicals Cf. chemical agents classification

Classification of corrosive burns Cf. corrosive burns classification

Classification of chemical weapons Cf. chemical weapons classification

Classification of fires Cf. class of fire

Classification of civil rights Cf. civil rights

Climate The aggregate of the average atmospheric conditions that characterize the weather of a given area. Example: continental climate.
Cf. continental climate, equatorial climate, maritime climate, monsoon climate, mountain climate, macroclimate

Climate change An identifiable change in the state of the climate that persists for a long time, over decades, caused either by natural phenomena or due to human activity – after IPCC.
Cf. climate, climatic control

Climate impact assessment An investigative practice for identifying and evaluating the harmful as well as beneficial consequences of climate change on natural, living and human systems – after IPCC.

Climatic control The complex of climatic factors that relatively permanently determine the general characteristics of the climate in a given region of the earth.
Cf. climate

Climatic zone Wide region of the earth sharing a generally similar climate, along the same latitudes, limited by mountains, plains, bodies of water and other atmospheric factors.
Cf. climatic region

Climatography Numerical presentation of the components of a region's climate by the use of maps, charts, graphs, models, diagrams, texts, etc.

Climatological forecast Forecast based on studies of the climate of a region and not on the dynamic consequences of the current weather. (Not to be confused with weather forecast.)
Cf. weather forecast

Climatology The study of climates, including the statistical average variation, distribution and frequencies of the meteorological elements.

Climigration A new term to describe forced permanent migration of communities due to severe climatic changes that impact on such infra-structures as schools, health clinics, livelihoods and well-being, e.g. seen recently in arctic regions – Bronen.

Clinical trials Scientific studies outside the laboratory through which the benefits of one or more medical therapies are assessed. The persons involved must give consent.

Cluster A group of similar things; or a natural grouping of persons, such as those of the same age, or the same sex; or a village in a district, in a refugee camp or other community. Convenient for statistics, administration or health programmes.
Cf. cohort

Cluster bomb A bomb that contains, and on impact disperses, more than 600 bomblets, which in turn explode over a wide perimeter, causing enormous damage directly. Up to 10–40% of the bombs or bomblets may not explode immediately and lie on or beneath the surface of the ground, secondarily exploding upon contact and causing further civilian injuries years after the cessation of hostilities. Many millions of cluster bombs still lie in open fields, unexploded, e.g. in Vietnam or in Southern Lebanon. The Oslo Treaty (2008) internationally prohibits their production, sale or use, but several States still unashamedly use or produce and sell them. Also known as fragmentation bombs.
Cf. fragmentation bomb, landmines, antipersonnel mines, Oslo Treaty

CNN effect Following news of a disaster situation or humanitarian crisis, the rise or fall in international awareness, interest and funding that fluctuate with the extent and duration of news media coverage.

Sn: CNN factor, media factor

Coast Shoreline of variable contours where the land, sea and atmosphere meet, with consequent environmental, social and economic influences.
Sn: littoral

Coccidioidomycosis A fungal infection due to inhalation of a soil fungus in dusty desert areas. Endemic in arid regions, particularly of the American continent.

Code of Conduct in Disaster Relief Cf. Disaster relief code of conduct

CODESEDH Spanish acronym for Committee for the Defence of Health, Professional Ethics and Human Rights, important humanitarian organization in Argentina and Latin America for human rights, especially against torture.
Cf. torture, ethics, human rights

Code share In the aviation industry, an agreement between airlines whereby a flight or other service is published with the codes of two or more airlines and the flight is operated by one of the participating carriers.
Cf. chartering

Codex Alimentarius/CA Jointly run by FAO and WHO, the CA Commission sets international food safety, production, quality and handling standards to protect the health of consumers and ensure fair practices in the national and international food trade.

Coefficient of tide The relation, at a given place, between the tidal range and the mean tidal range during a defined period.
Cf. tide

Cohort A group of persons of the same age group banded together or recruited into a population at the same time. Age class.
Cf. age profile, cluster

Cold chain System of refrigeration with appropriate apparatus and transport facilities to ensure the cold or frozen conservation of vaccines, blood, medicaments and tissues throughout the transfer, from the place of manufacture and expedition to the point of arrival and use.

For the blood cold chain the term "from vein to vein" is used.

Cf. vaccine, Expanded Programme on Immunization, refrigeration

Cold front thunderstorm Type of thunderstorm which occurs in series along a cold front or along a line that precedes a cold front.

Cf. thunderstorm

Coliform bacilli The various bacteria which are normal inhabitants of the intestines but which become pathogenic under certain conditions. *E. coli* is the commonest.

Cf. diarrhoeal diseases, enteric diseases

Collateral damage Injury to persons or damage to property inflicted unintentionally following the use of a weapon, a nuclear explosion, other attack or harmful event.

Cf. transboundary pollution, fallout, acceptable collateral damage

Collective dose In a nuclear accident or war, the total dose of radiation to an exposed population, expressed as the product of the mean individual dose by the total number of persons exposed.

Cf. absorbed dose, dose, maximum acceptable dose, retained dose

Colonization/Colonialism Microbiology: The setting and multiplication of microorganisms on a host species or bacteriological medium.

Politics: The claiming of alien lands forcefully, settling people and a foreign government on such lands, thus colonizing the country and exercising power and activities usually with primary consideration for their own benefits rather than the interests of the host (colonized) population. Colonialism, with colonies and colonial empires, was part of international power politics from the eighteenth to the twentieth century, with a dominant's psychology of the powerful colonizer and depressed reaction of the colonized. Most colonies gained freedom in the mid-twentieth century.

Command and control A term and system borrowed from the military which relates to the organization, coordination, process and control of all stages and methods of activities to ensure the successful management of a disaster or other major event.

Commission of European Communities The institutional arrangements bringing together the European Communities with the aim of gradually integrating their economies and moving towards political unity, with a European Parliament in Brussels. The name has been changed to European Union (EU). Has an active programme (Echo) for disaster relief and assistance to developing countries and civil protection.

Sn: European Union

Cf. Council of Europe, ECHO

Commodity rate In transportation, special low rates applicable in air freight traffic for certain categories of supplies, e.g. emergency medicines, between designated airports of origin and destination.

Sn: concessionary rate

Common source outbreak A disease outbreak that results from a group of persons being exposed to the same common agent.

Communal dwelling A housing estate, usually multistorey, sharing common areas (entrance, stairs, etc.) and services (heating, caretaking) built to house a considerable number of people.
Cf. dwelling, services

Communal facilities All the physical infrastructure and the social and cultural facilities needed for the collective life of a community.
Cf. community

Communicable disease An infectious condition that can be transmitted from one living person or animal to another person or animal through a variety of channels, according to the nature of the disease.
Sn: infectious disease, contagious disease
Cf. contagious period

Communicable period Period during which an infectious agent can be transmitted directly or indirectly from one person or animal to another person or animal. Sn: contagious period, transmissible period
Cf. carrier, infection

Communication resources Inventory of all public and private communication facilities: police, fire, military, government, private radio, amateur (HAM) radio operators, newspapers, other news media, television, telephone and telex, Internet, social network, satellite and other facilities that can be used in time of disaster

Community The complex of individuals or groups of varying size sharing common values, interests or problems, within a given area. Examples: neighbourhood community, rural community, European community.

Community health worker A health worker, male or female, chosen by the community and usually living in the community, trained to deal with the health problems of his community and its individuals and to work in close relationship with the health services. CHWs provide the first contact between the individual and health system – WHO.
Cf. primary health care, community

Complex disaster/Complex Emergency A major disaster or complicated emergency situation affecting large civilian populations, which is further aggravated by intense political and/or military interferences, including war or civil strife, resulting in serious food shortage, epidemics, population displacements, poverty, loss of human liberties and significant increase in mortality, rendering the management of the situation very complex. Breakdown of government infrastructures hampers humanitarian aid. Examples: Afghanistan, Rwanda, Somalia. (Not to be confused with compound disaster.)
Cf. compound disaster, disaster

Complex Emergencies Database CE-DAT, a compilation by CRED that provides information on health, nutrition mortality and epidemiology in complex humanitarian emergencies.
Cf. EM-DAT, Centre for Research in Epidemiology of Disasters, complex emergencies, compound emergencies

Complexity theory An approach for transforming the chaotic and complicated into something understandable and simpler. A theory according to which a large number of seemingly independent agents can be made to spontaneously organize themselves into a coherent, less complex system.

Cf. chaos theory, catastrophe theory

Compound disaster A disaster where the concurrent occurrence of more than one kind of major emergency at the same time and place magnifies, aggravates and compounds the destructive event. Example, the 2011 disaster in Japan represented an earthquake, a tsunami, a nuclear reactor failure and a great number of deaths, all taking place on 11 March and in the same region, compounding the seriousness and complication of the disaster. (Not to be confused with complex disaster, where the political, conflict and military elements are predominant factors.) – Gunn.

Cf. complex disaster

Concentration at ground level The degree of concentration of a pollutant in the air, measured from ground level up to an adult person's height.

Sn: ground level concentration

Concentration camp A supervised and controlled area, provided with buildings, huts or tents and other minimal facilities, reserved for the accommodation of political prisoners, prisoners of war, internees and other victims and persons or groups that the authorities wish to keep under control. Some concentration camps, such as Auschwitz, have been notoriously brutal death camps, against all humanitarian law.

Cf. prison, prisoner of war, Auschwitz, pogrom

Concessionary rate Sn: commodity rate

Conciliation Cf. arbitration

Concrete encasement Rendering completely and definitively out of commission a nuclear facility, such as the damaged reactor in Chernobyl, by

totally and hermetically covering/sealing it in heavily reinforced concrete, known as a sarcophagus. However, with time, cracks, wear and leakages, the expected safety has failed, and a new steel sarcophagus is being constructed. A continuous disaster.

Cf. Chernobyl, sarcophagus, nuclear activity, reactor

Concussion A relatively mild, temporary mental alteration, with or without loss of consciousness, following head injury.

Conditioning Psychophysiological mechanism, and techniques, of associations between a simple or complex stimulus and an unconscious act.

Confidentiality The principle and practice of ensuring and maintaining the privacy and security of any information obtained in trust from or concerning a person or institution in the privileged circumstances of a hierarchical, personal or professional relationship.

Conflagration Fire: any great, serious and destructive fire.

In nuclear war, the propagation of fires by the wind, following the coalescence of separate fires ignited by the explosion's thermal pulse, or blast wave – Rotblat.

Cf. fireball, firestorm, nuclear war, superfires

Conflict A general term for any military, political or ideological struggle, armed or otherwise; personal group opposition, antagonism or clash; declared or undeclared hostilities, civil war, fighting within a state or between one or more enemy countries. If undeclared or international, the instruments of International Humanitarian Law of the United Nations may have difficulty to apply.

Cf. armed conflict, war, Geneva Conventions, International Humanitarian Law, United Nations

Conflict diamonds The illegal practice of certain warlords, kleptocrats and unethical financiers to provide funds for wars and conflicts, especially in Africa, through the illicit sale of diamonds. Measures of international certification of diamonds are introduced (Kimberley Process) to counteract such sales. Also referred to as blood diamonds.
Cf. blood diamonds, Kimberley Process, conflict, kleptocracy

Conscientious objector Person who on moral grounds and personal conscience refuses, rejects, objects to undertaking certain actions, especially military service. In some tolerant countries, such release from military service may be supplanted by useful social service.

Consent General: Voluntarily giving one's agreement or permission to a proposed plan, complying with another person's expressed desire or concurring with a plan of action.
Health care: All treatment or experimentation must have the patient's informed consent. Forced declarations, unconsented experiments, undesired treatment or actions are not permitted.
Cf. Nuremberg Code, Helsinki Declaration

Consignment In transport and shipping, a certain amount of cargo, defined by one transport document, where its weight, size, number of parcels or appearance are stated.

Consolidation In transport and shipping, the assembling of several loads originating from several sources for joint dispatch.

Contact case Person living in proximity to a contagious patient likely or suspected to have been contaminated and possible to suffer or transmit the disease, thus necessitating surveillance and prophylactic measures.
Cf. carrier, communicable period, contamination, surveillance

Contagious period Sn: communicable period

Container A standard shipping metallic box, of steel or aluminium, with double doors at one end, in use on sea routes, for easier handling and safe transportation of cargo. There are two types: the 20-ft container, 30 m^3 capacity, 18 tons load and the 40 ft, 60 m^3 capacity, 30 tons load. Discarded containers have at times been transformed and used as dwellings in disaster or refugee areas.
Cf. crate

Contamination
1. Invasion of a person or animal by pathogenic germs (contaminants).
2. Presence of an infectious agent on inanimate articles such as clothes, surgical instruments, dressings, water, milk, food.
3. Undesirable presence of a radioactive material.
4. Transfer or propagation of a contaminant.
Cf. infection, radioactive contamination

Continental anticyclone Anticyclone situated over a continent during the cold season, caused mainly by prolonged cooling of the earth's surface and by low temperatures in the lower layers of the atmosphere.
Cf. anticyclone

Continental climate The typical climate of the interior of continents characterized by the large annual or daily amplitude of the temperature.
Cf. climate

Continental erosion Disintegration, in every form, of the soil through the effect of atmospheric agents: frost, dripping, wind, temperature variations, chemical reactions, streaming. Cf. erosion, wind

Continental shelf The submarine continuation of the margins of the continent extending beneath the sea at a gentle slope.

Contingency plan An anticipatory emergency plan to be followed in an expected or eventual disaster, based on risk assessment, availability of human and material resources, community preparedness, local and international response capability, etc.
Sn: emergency plan
Cf. disaster plan, plan

Contribution Material or financial aid to an organization or country, without compensation expected from the recipient.
Sn: donation
Cf. aid, donor, recipient

Contribution in kind Assistance in case of disaster that consists of materials (e.g. tents, pharmaceuticals) or services (e.g. experts, transport) but not of monetary donations or financial help.
Sn: in-kind contribution
Cf. relief

Conurbation The comprehensive system composed of a town and its extensions, with suburbs, shopping centre, station, green spaces, etc.
Cf. urbanization

Convective thunderstorm Thunderstorm that accompanies a convective cloud, especially when such a cloud is caused by local conditions, such as forest fires.

Convention refugee Person who meets the definition of Article I of the 1951 UN Convention relative to the status of refugees.

Cf. refugee, refugee protection, UNHCR

Conventional arms/weapons Arms, weapons or forces that are nonnuclear, non-biological, non-chemical, such as conventional guns, tanks, battleships, aircraft, troops, etc. Whence conventional defence, conventional forces. They are the opposite of arms/weapons of mass destruction.
Cf. weapons of mass destruction

Conventional food Food available or obtained through the traditional methods of agriculture, animal husbandry, hunting, fishing, gathering or cooking within the community and not subjected to unconventional, foreign processing methods.
Cf. bulghur, cassava, sorghum, yam, yoghourt

Convergence in disasters A common phenomenon in disaster situations, people moving in many different directions but converging in mainly two different ways: (1) internal convergence: towards hospitals, casualty points, rescue centres, morgue, television stations; (2) external convergence: aid suppliers, NGOs, disaster responders, the press, etc. Proper management of these divers' movements is important.

Copenhagen Declaration The World Summit for Social Development, gathered in Copenhagen in 1995, studied and declared the broad range of social services, political, economic cultural health, institutional and other factors that retard or influence social development, especially under changing forces of globalization that often bypass the state. The Copenhagen Declaration contains ten Commitments:
(1) Enabling environment for social development, (2) peradication, (3)

full employment and secure and sustainable livelihoods, (4) social integration, (5) gender equity, (6) basic services and promotion of culture, (7) accelerated development of Africa and least developed countries, (8) social dimensions in structural environment, (9) increased revenues for social development.

The follow-up World Summit for Social Development and Beyond – Achieving Social Development for All in a Globalizing World met in Geneva in 2000 and endorsed and strengthened these Commitments.

Cf. development, socio-economic survey, MDGs

Coping capacity For a country, the coping capacity is the degree of preparedness and adaptation of its population, of its institutions and its physical readiness, depending on the available resources, plans and abilities.

At the individual level, on impact or following a disaster, some persons demonstrate an acute stress reaction, which is a severe but rapidly transient episode in otherwise healthy conditions. Not all persons suffer such a disorder, as they have a better biological and mental response capacity. Increased coping capacity may also be demonstrated by groups or populations, amounting to resilience.

Cf. disaster preparedness, adaptability, resilience, burn out, post-traumatic stress

Cor Unum Cf. Caritas Internationalis

Corium In a nuclear reactor accident, designates the melted nuclear and metallic material that remains in the tanks.

Cf. nuclear accident

Corn-soya blend A nutritional mixture made up of:

69.7% cornmeal, processed, gelatinized
22% soya flour, defatted, toasted
5.5% soya oil, refined, deodorized, stabilized
2.7% mineral premix
0.1% vitamin antioxidant premix
Sn: CSB
Cf. food mixtures

Corn-soya-milk A nutritional mixture made up of:

59.2% cornmeal, processed, gelatinized
17.5% soya flour, defatted, toasted
15% non-fat dry milk, spray processed
5.5% soya oil, refined, deodorized, stabilized
2.7% mineral premix
0.1% vitamin, antioxidant premix
Sn: CSM
Cf. food mixtures

Corrosion

1. Burns: Synonym for chemical burn. The chemical agents that cause burns can be basically divided into alkalis and acids. Other agents are phosphorus and blister forming (mainly war) gases.
   Cf. chemical burns.

2. Metallurgy: The gradual destruction or rusting of a metal or alloy due to oxidation and action of chemicals, causing weakness and metal fatigue that may result in equipment failure or building collapse.

Corruption Morally contemptible, unethical and socially unacceptable acts by commission or omission with the view to illegally obtaining and amassing, property, position, favours, false statements, advancement and wealth, mainly by extortion, coercion and undemocratic ways, in exchange of bribes, power, promotion, money,

personal favours, threats and unlawful actions. Very unfortunately, such
condemnable acts are common and
institutionalized in some countries or
governments that have no concern
for the real needs of their people and
constitute causes of poverty and
underdevelopment.

Cf. kleptocracy, deontology, ethics,
Transparency International, man-conceived disaster

Cosmic radiation Beams of very high
energy particles (protons, alpha
particles and certain heavier nuclei)
of solar, galactic or extragalactic
origin.

Cf. ionizing radiation

Cost-benefit Cf. cost-benefit analysis

Cost-benefit analysis
1. Study of the various elements of a
situation in order to determine the
feasibility of an aid or action
2. Methods to compare alternatives of
the price (costs) and advantages
(benefits) of an operation in monetary
terms with the view to determining
the most desirable course of action.

Cf. cost-effectiveness analysis

Cost-effectiveness analysis A method
of evaluation of programmes whereby
the costs are quantified in monetary
terms and the advantages in non-
monetary terms of effectiveness in
relation to the desired goal.

Cf. cost-benefit analysis, goal

Council of Europe Organization bringing together, at Strasbourg, all the
States of Europe, to "achieve a greater
unity for the purpose of safeguarding
and realizing the ideals and principles
which are their common heritage and
facilitating their economic and social
progress". Not to confuse with the
European Union. Promotes the
European Centre for Disaster Medicine, human rights.

Sn: CE

Cf. European Centre for Disaster
Medicine, European Union

**Council on Health Research for
Development/COHRED** Govern-
ment-aided, non-profit international
organization that promotes and
facilitates health research, especially in developing countries, with
priority for diseases in the poorest
countries.

Cf. ten/ninety gap

Counterfeit drugs Medicaments that
are fraudulently manufactured, or
illegally mislabelled or mispackaged
or fake concerning their origin and
pharmacology, sold for gain and not
for health benefits. Dangerous.

Counterforce attack Nuclear weapons
deployed against the enemy's military installations, as distinct from
economic and industrial targets.

Cf. countervalue attack, nuclear war

Countervalue attack Nuclear weapons
deployed against the enemy's
industrial and economic potential, as
distinct from its military bases.

Cf. counterforce attack, nuclear war

Country economic profile Economic categorization of countries by the World
Bank according to their gross national
income, GNI (previously GNP, gross
national product). For 2008 the grouping is (a) low-income countries: US$975
or less, (b) lower-middle income:
US$976–3,855, (c) upper-middle
income: US$ 3,856–11,905, (d) higher
income: US$11,906 or more.

Country health profile Summary
description of a country's existing
morbidity; mortality; endemic diseases; chronic conditions; nutritional
state; demographic profile; health
facilities as hospitals, outpatient clinics, health centres, pharmacies, mother
and child facilities, care delivery

systems, ambulances; health resources, as physicians, nurses, primary health care personnel. May include Ministry of Health budget.

Country of asylum Country which offers some protection to a person who has fled his country of origin, of nationality or of usual residence.
Cf. asylum, protection of refugees, territorial asylum

Country of first asylum The first country where a refugee arrives and receives asylum after having left his own country.
Cf. refugee, territorial asylum

Country of second asylum Country, other than that of first asylum, that accepts a refugee for asylum and settlement.
Cf. asylum, country of first asylum, refugee, territorial asylum

Covenant A binding agreement. In international relations, it is often used for a treaty.
Cf. treaty

Cranfield Mine Action A unit at Cranfield University, UK, that supports UN and governmental activities in research, management and training for the improvement of anti-mine action.
Cf. mines, antipersonnel mines, Ottawa Treaty, Geneva Centre for Humanitarian Demining

Crate In transport or shipping, open case made of planks assembled, nailed and strapped, which show contents or their inner packing, as opposed to a closed case.
Cf. container

Crater The bowl-shaped cavity due to the eruption of a volcano, to an explosion or to impact. Usually the mouth of a volcano.

Creep In earthquake, science creep refers to the fault displacement that occurs as slow aseismic slip, as in the San Andreas fault in California. It is not clear whether changes in creep may be associated with earthquake precursors.
In disastrology, a creeping disaster refers to a slow-onset disaster, as in drought leading to famine.

Creeping disaster A disaster of insidious onset and slow progress, such as famine, drought, desertification, health deterioration or epidemic, that does not become manifest until damage and suffering reach extensive proportions in numbers and gravity and need massive emergency response.
There is also a kind of creeping earthquake.
Sn: slow onset disaster

Creutzfeldt-Jakob disease Subacute spongiform encephalopathy. A slow brain infection with progressive visual disturbances, dementia, neuromuscular disequilibrium (ataxia) and death. Caused by a new class of infectious agents close to proteins, called prions. It is a human variant of mad cow disease and bovine spongiform encephalopathy. Can spread in epidemic proportions by ingestion of infected meat, especially beef.
Sn: human spongiform encephalopathy
Cf. mad cow disease, prion, BSE, zoonosis

Crime of aggression In its revision of the Treaty of Rome the Kampala Conference of 2010 as well as the Princeton Process have defined "crime of aggression" for the International Criminal Court. The UN Charter defines it as "the gravest …unlawful use of force".
Cf. aggression, crime of

Crimes against humanity Crimes concerning the international community as a whole, carried out in widespread and/or systematic manner, and/or on

a massive scale and/or on specified grounds, in war or peacetime. According to the International Criminal Court, they include any of the following acts committed as part of a widespread or systematic attack directed against any civilian population, with knowledge of the attack: (a) murder; (b) extermination; (c) enslavement; (d) deportation or forcible transfer of population; (e) imprisonment or other deprivation of physical liberty; (f) torture; (g) rape, sexual slavery, enforced prostitution, enforced sterilization or any other comparable sexual violence; (h) persecution against any identifiable group on political, racial, national, ethnic, cultural, religious, gender or other grounds universally impermissible; (i) enforced disappearance of persons; (j) crime of apartheid; (k) other inhumane acts of similar character intentionally causing suffering – ICT. Such crimes are punishable by International Law.
Cf. human rights, extermination, genocide, International Criminal Court, man-conceived disaster, concentration camp, Universal Declaration of Human Rights

Crisis From the Greek krinò, decide; a low probability but high-consequent, crucial event, usually a harmful turning point, a dangerous and critical moment of decision in management, commerce, war, law, illness, personal or social relations that poses a grave challenge and requires immediate action.
Cf. crisis management, coping capacity

Crisis management The art, managerial skills, preparedness, provision of facilities, leadership capacity for rapid decisions, to assemble all required aids and act appropriately at the right moment with the view to an appropriate solution, damage control or disaster response.
Cf. Health Action in Crises (WHO)

Crisis relocation Due to a disaster or other critical necessity, the planned and orderly evacuation and siting of individuals or populations to a safer and more appropriate area. This should under no circumstances be a deportation.
Cf. deportation, resettlement

Critical facilities The primary physical structures, technical facilities and systems which are socially, economically or operationally essential to the functioning of a society or community, both in routine circumstances and in the extreme circumstances of an emergency – UNISDR.

Critical pathway(s) In management, a road map or outline of step-by-step actions and processes to be followed to best achieve the desired goal.

Crop rotation Cultivation of successive different crops on the same land, over a number of seasons, in order to maintain the fertility of the soil.

Cross-cultural study An investigation and documentation in which populations from different cultural backgrounds in a given area are compared.

Crowd A multiple of persons fortuitously or voluntarily gathered in a particular place, with or without any obvious organization. Crowds can become an additional riot problem in disaster situations.

Crush syndrome A severe, life-threatening trauma caused by an extensive compression (crushing), e.g. by entrapment under rubble in an earthquake, resulting in massive destruction of muscle and bone, bleeding,

fluid loss, with release of toxins (myoglobin) in the circulation and kidney damage.
Cf. emergency medical services, trauma scale, shock

Cultural relativism A view according to which cultural differences should be taken into account and interpreted differently when certain principles (such as the fundamental values of human rights) are considered in different cultures. A doctrine that is opposed to the principle of universality of values, e.g. that all human rights are held by all persons and cultures without distinction, and makes way to differences.
Cf. Universal Declaration of Human Rights

Culture A combination of beliefs, traditions, customs, myths, practices, moral values, religious obligations and intellectual qualities that are associated with or recognized as the heritage of a group of people, citizens of a country or members of a national or ethnic community.

Cumulative effect The progressive increase, by summation, of the effects of an external agent on an organism, an individual or society.

Custom The usual way of doing things, behaving, reacting in face of a particular situation or appearing according to a tradition. In jurisprudence, custom is established usage having the force of law. Expatriate disaster responders must respect local customs and traditions even under emergency conditions, as directed by standard No. 5 of the Code of Conduct in Disaster Relief.
Cf. customary law, Code of conduct in disaster relief

Customary Law Customs that have been so much associated with a particular population or country and have been in practice for so long that they

have become binding and part of codified law.
In international law, customary law refers to the law of nations.
Cf. custom

Cyanide Hydrogen cyanide and cyanogen chloride, called blood gas, lethal chemical weapons.
Cf. chemical warfare, Geneva Protocol, WMD, CBW

Cyberwar The use of secret electronic computer-based viruses intruding from a distance in the opponent's military, economic or other competing system, by hackers intercepting, making it unusable or destroying it, e.g. Stuxnet.
Cf. Stuxnet, star wars, hacking, Strategic Defense Initiative

Cyclone A storm characterized by the converging and rising gyratory movement of the wind around a zone of low pressure (the eye) towards which it is violently pulled from a zone of high pressure. Its circulation is counterclockwise round the centre in the northern hemisphere, clockwise in the southern hemisphere.
Cf. non-tropical cyclone, tropical cyclone, hurricane, typhoon, Beaufort scale, Saffir-Simpson scale

Cyclone   warning Meteorological message intended to warn the population concerned of the existence or approach of a cyclone. It may be accompanied by advice on protective measures to take.

Cyclonic rain In the classification of rainfall, it denotes a violent heavy and continuous rain whose minimal intensity is rarely below 5–10 mm/h. The two other classes are "orographic" and "convective" rain.

Cysticercosis An intestinal helminth infection caused by the larvae (cysticerci) of *Taenia solium* (pork tapeworm) which also attacks the muscles.

Sn: tapeworm infection, taeniasis
Cy. neglected tropical disease, zoonosis

D

DALE/DALY Acronyms for disability adjusted life expectancy and disability adjusted life years (Cf.)

Dag Hammerskjöld Library/UN The principal United Nations Library in New York, depository of all the documents, reports, publications in all the spheres of the UN and specialized agencies and other publications in the international field.

Dam A strong barrier structure built across a river basin to retain, divert or control the flow for such purposes as water supply, navigation, power production, flood control, irrigation. The resulting changes may have important socio-economic and environmental consequences.

Damage assessment/analysis Detailed evaluation and determination of the actual damages caused by a disaster.
Sn: damage analysis
Cf. damage forecasting, damage probability formula

Damage classification Evaluation and recording of damage to the built environment, structures, objects or facilities according to categories.

1. "Severe damage": damage that precludes further use of the structure, facility or object for its intended purpose.
2. "Moderate damage": degree of damage to principal members that would preclude effective use of the structure, facility, or object for its intended use, unless major repairs were made short of complete reconstruction.

3. "Light damage", such as broken window, slight damage to roof and siding, interior partitions blown down and cracked walls; the damage not being severe enough to preclude use of installation for the purpose for which it was intended – OFDA.
Cf. damage assessment

Damage control Cf. damage mitigation, crisis management

Damage forecasting Study made prior to a disaster, of the situation, expected or eventual damage and probable effects of different types of disaster.;
Cf. damage assessment, disaster preparedness

Damage mitigation Decisions and measures taken to attenuate or lessen the extent of damage, of hardship and of suffering caused by disaster.
Cf. disaster mitigation, crisis management

Damage probability formula

$$P_D = f(P_H)(H_{man} + H_{nat})(R_H)$$
$$(V_{nat} + a_1 + a_2 + b_1 + b_2)$$

where: P is the probability, D is the damage or disaster;
P_D is the probability that an event will inflict damage on the society or environment at risk;
H is hazard;
R_H is the probability (risk) that this hazard will be converted into an event;
f is a function of the relationship between all the variables contained within and between the brackets;
P_H is the probability of an event occurring that may result in damage;

H_{man} is the human component responsible for the hazard to exist;

H_{nat} is hazard as given by nature;

V is vulnerability;

V_{nat} is the natural vulnerability;

a is the sum of the actions before an event occurs;

a_1 is the augmentation of vulnerability;

a_2 is mitigation of vulnerability;

b is the sum of the actions taken during or after an event occurs;

b_1 is counterproductive disaster response;

b_2 is the productive, alleviatory disaster response.

(The term *f* for function must be considered as a *generic* mathematical entity, not meant as a quantitative statement.)

The ultimate objective of disaster management is to bring the probability that damage will occur (P_D) as close to zero as possible – WADEM.

Cf. damage assessment, damage forecasting, damage mitigation, human failure, Utstein, WADEM

De facto refugee A term used for two categories of persons:

(a) Persons who fulfil the requirements of a refugee definition but who, for various reasons, such as a procedural delay in submitting the application within a specified time, have not been registered as refugees.

(b) Persons who cannot prove a justified fear of persecution within the meaning of refugee definition, but who are considered, on similar grounds, to have valid reasons for not wishing to return to their country of origin.

Cf. refugee

De jure refugee Sn: statutory refugee; Cf. refugee

Death rate The ratio between the number of deaths in a given time and the total number of the population.; Sn: mortality rate

Debris flow A flow of dense concentration of mud, rocks, trees, construction remains and refuse, carried downwards.

Cf. mud flow

Decedent Person who has died. A dead individual.

Deck cargo In transport and shipping, under deck cargo means goods stowed inside the holds of a vessel; on deck cargo means goods stowed above the holds "on deck", on the vessel, mostly because of their hazardous nature. On deck cargo will be the first to be jettisoned in case of emergency. Deck goods are always carried without any acceptance of responsibility by the carrier.

Declaration of disaster Official announcement made by the competent authorities declaring a state of emergency in the wake of a disaster and the need for special measures to cope with it. Certain donor countries and organizations cannot provide assistance unless a disaster has been officially declared by the stricken country and aid requested.

Cf. request for disaster assistance

Decontamination Bacteriology: Reducing the microbial presence and infection capacity to a safe level.; Nuclear: In the context of radiation contamination, all the physical and other measures taken to reduce radiation activity in terms of physical quantity, activity of waste and the radionuclide content.

Defibrillator A device that sends a strong electric charge to the myocardium, thus stimulating conduction tissue and restoring regular sinus rhythm to a heart in fibrillation or that has ceased to beat – Last.

Deficiency disease A general term that denotes physiological dysfunction due to the lack or insufficiency of a number of factors needed to ensure health and well-being. It may be due to lack of nutritional factors (nutritional deficiency, protein energy deficiency, vitamin deficiency), biological (iron deficiency, iodine deficiency), immunological deficiency (genetic or acquired), etc.

When not specified and especially in disaster situations, the term usually denotes nutritional deficiency.

Sn: deficiency syndrome

Cf. vitamin deficiency, goitre

Deflation The removal and erosion of soil by the wind.

Defoliant Chemical compound used as pesticide, especially against plant pests. Also used as a weapon in chemical warfare.

Cf. chemical warfare, pesticide, agent orange

Deforestation Destruction of forests or the clearing of an area of its trees and undergrowth, which can lead to a major deterioration of the environmental conditions, such as soil erosion, disturbance of the water table and catchment areas, scarcity of animal life, temperature changes, etc.

Cf. catchment basin, environment, erosion, soil erosion

Degree of adaptability The relative ability of a living organism, of a society or of a population to adapt to unfavourable changes in the environment.

Cf. adaptation, environment

Dehydration Depletion of the body's water and fluid reserves, with disturbances of cellular salts, due to excessive fluid loss (diarrhoea, vomiting, heavy perspiration, fever) or insufficient intake (drought, malnutrition), or metabolic disease or a combination of these, causing cell damage, particularly serious in infants and in debilitated persons. A 10–15% water deficit constitutes moderate to severe dehydration. The maximum degree of loss compatible with life is about 20%. Provision of fluids and rehydration salts is vital.

Cf. cholera, diarrhoea, rehydration salts, water

Delegate

1. Representative of an international organization in a foreign country.
2. Title of the expert representative of the International Committee of the Red Cross.

Cf. representative

Delirium An acute state of confusion, usually a consequence of intoxication by drugs, alcohol or other substances. May also accompany a high degree of fever, especially in children.

Delta Triangular configuration of a section of coast open to the sea, created by the alluvial deposits at the mouth of a river, often – but not always – traversed by its branches. Example: the Nile delta.

Cf. alluvium, mouth

Democracy From the Greek demos=people, and kratein=rule. Rule by the people, as opposed to rule by a person or autocrat. The form of government in which the sovereign power resides in the people, with equal rights for all, and exercised by free vote through their representatives.

Cf. autocrat, dictator

Democratic Control of Armed Forces/ Geneva Centre for A Swiss-led international foundation in Geneva with mission to assist the international community in pursuance of good governance and reform of the security sector by developing norms and standards, conducting policy research, promoting the rule of law and supporting democratic security governance.
Sn: DCAF

Demographic concentration The establishment of a population over a given territory.
Sn: population concentration

Demography The quantitative study of human populations and of their variations.

Demurrage In transportation and storage, the rent in railway sheds. Penalty for keeping containers longer than allowed. Penalty for immobilization of a vessel longer than allowed for loading/unloading and payable by owners of the goods.

Dengue An acute febrile illness of sudden onset, with headache, fever, prostration, swollen glands, joint and muscle ache and skin rash. Transmitted through the mosquito, it can cause epidemics in displaced settlements. A more serious form is dengue haemorrhagic fever. A neglected tropical disease.
Sn: dengue fever
Cf. dengue haemorrhagic fever, neglected tropical disease

Dengue haemorrhagic fever A severe form of dengue with sudden fever, bleeding and collapse, often fatal. Prevalent in Southeast Asia and India.
Cf. dengue

Denial Cf. rejection

Density factor The ratio of the concentration of a radionuclide in an organism (organ or tissue) to the concentration of that radionuclide in the environment.
Cf. radionuclide, maximum acceptable concentration

Denudation
1. Geology: Stripping or laying bare of rocks by removal of the topping soil or other ground cover.
Sn: stripping.
2. Medicine: Exposing a vein for intravenous infusion, e.g. for fluid loss.
Sn: cut-down

Deontology The study and application of a particular profession's ethics – in this case, the ethics and correct practices of the medical profession, disaster managers and the law.

Deoxyribonucleic acid/DNA The molecule that carries the genetic information for most living systems.
Sn: DNA
Cf. chromosome

Dependence Social: The situation of relying on someone else and needing personal support.
Societal: A community, e.g. refugees, flood victims, or a government depending on outside aid.
Medical: An addicted person dependent on drugs. Sn: substance abuse.

Depopulation A fall in the population of a region due to (a) emigration or (b) an excess of deaths over births.
Cf. birth rate, death rate, emigration

Deportation The forcible transfer of a population, forced displacement of the persons concerned by expulsion or other coercive acts, from the area where they are lawfully present, without grounds permitted under international law – ICC.
Cf. civil rights, human rights, International Criminal Court, UDHR, disappearance, genocide

Depression

1. Atmosphere/climatology: Centre of an atmospheric pressure which is low in relation to the surrounding region at the same level. It is characterized by high winds that increase towards the centre and blow mainly anticlockwise in the northern hemisphere.
   Sn: non-tropical cyclone
   Cf. cyclone
2. Psychology: A state of gloominess, sadness, dejection, low spirits.
3. Economics: A period marked by _ business downturn, high unemployment, low wages, gloomy finances. Its persistence and worsening may lead to an economic disaster.

Desert Region characterized by excessive dryness (WMO dryness ratio greater than 10), too little rainfall, extremely poor vegetation, no arable land, shifting sand, very sparse population and particularly difficult living conditions.
Cf. desertification, drought, famine

Desertification Processes whereby a semi-arid ecosystem loses the capacity of seasonal revival or repair and progresses towards becoming desert. As a result of climatic factors and human activity (excessive grazing, deforestation, bush fires, etc.), there is increase of bare soil, decrease of vegetation-covered soil, rise in reflection of solar light, excessive to permanent loss of plant life, soil erosion and impoverishment. Such degradation causes environmental damage well beyond its boundaries and is itself a combined natural and man-made disaster.
Cf. desert, drought, famine, savannah, semi-arid zone, Sahel

Developing country A country where the economic indicators show low levels of industrialization, low gross national income (GNI, previously GDP), low literacy rate, health levels, life expectancy, students per capita and low levels of investment and saving.
Cf. country economic categories, development, emerging countries

Development A comprehensive economic, social, cultural and political process which aims at the constant improvement and well-being of the entire population and of individuals on the basis of their actions, free meaningful participation in development and in the fair distribution of benefits therefrom – UN: The Right to Development.
Cf. sustainable development, Millennium Development Goals, sustainable development

Development Assistance Research Associates/DARA An independent NGO based in Spain and Switzerland devoted to the effectiveness and quality of developmental aid to vulnerable populations affected by conflict, disaster or climate change. Provides objective quality analysis and evaluation of humanitarian operations and contributes to the improvement of donor assistance according to its Humanitarian Response Index and Good Humanitarian Donorship aims.
Sn: DARA International
Cf. good humanitarian donorship, humanitarian response index, HRI, international assistance, beneficiary, humanitarian charter

Deworming Eliminating pathological, infectious worms from the intestinal tract by the oral administration of appropriate medicines.

Diamonds (corruption) Cf. blood diamonds, conflict diamonds, Kimberley Process, kleptocracy

Diarrhoea Increased fluidity, frequency and volume of bowel movements per day. Usually endemic in developing countries, it can rise to alarming proportions, with dehydration, in unsanitary or disaster situations. Passing at least three liquid stools a day is generally considered to constitute diarrhoea.
Cf. diarrhoeal diseases, oral rehydration

Diarrhoeal diseases Common gastro-intestinal diseases caused by a variety of pathogenic agents – that most often remain unidentified – involving most often young, undernourished children, especially in developing countries. In disaster conditions, these diseases become more widespread and serious due to shortage of drinking water, lack of hygiene and insufficient food. Infantile diarrhoea is caused mainly by premature weaning and artificial feeding.
Cf. diarrhoea, hygiene, malnutrition, oral rehydration

Diaspora From the Greek, literally means dispersing the seed. The scattering of a large population from its usual, traditional habitat or country by massive departures, through socio-economic difficulties, coercion, persecution or deportation and dispersing or settling among other populations in other countries. Examples: the Irish diaspora in the United States, Ukrainians in Canada, Huguenots in South Africa, Armenians in France, Palestinians in the Middle East.
Cf. deportation, refugee, exodus, Universal Declaration of Human Rights

Diet The rational consumption of solid and liquid foods by a healthy or sick individual or by a population.

Dietetics The science and principles of food for the healthy and the sick person, with the aim of satisfying the energy and nutritional needs of the body.
Cf. health, needs, nutrition

Dioxin The chemical compound 2, 3, 7, 8, tetra chlorodibenzo-p-dioxin, an extremely toxic substance used in manufacturing some herbicides. The harmful effects are very persistent and capable of causing severe illness and chromosomal malformations. A major accident occurred in Seveso. Also known as TCDD.
Cf. transboundary pollution, Seveso, agent orange, man-made disaster, toxicological disaster

Diphtheria An acute contagious disease mainly of children, characterized by a fibrinous pseudomembrane on the nasopharynx and larynx. Transmitted usually by direct contact and preventable by immunization. One of the diseases in the WHO global vaccination programme.
Cf. contact case, communicable disease, Expanded Programme on Immunization, infectious disease, vaccination

Diplomatic asylum Asylum provided by a State in the premises of its embassy or diplomatic mission.
Cf. territorial asylum

Diplomatic personnel/immunity The heads and the personnel of an embassy, consulate (to a state) and diplomatic mission (to a UN agency), who by international convention enjoy diplomatic status, in particular personal inviolability, juridical immunity, tax exemption and free customs privileges. The diplomatic pouch cannot be inspected at customs crossings.

Diplomatic pouch/bag Official carrying bag of diplomatic personnel that by international convention can cross frontiers and enter countries, enjoying immunity and free from inspection.

Dirty bomb Bomb with usual explosive TNT content to which has been added radioactive material.

Disability Disability is a diminution of any kind in a person's ability or restriction or impairment in the performance of any activity that is generally considered normal within the manner or range of a human being. Such diminution may be temporary or permanent, of physical, mental, sensory or intellectual nature, congenital or acquired.

Disability-adjusted life expectancy/ Disability-adjusted life years
In the assessment of health systems and burden of disease, two advanced methods of measuring goal achievements are used: (a) DALE (Disability-adjusted life expectancy) is used to assess how well the objective of good health is being achieved; and (b) DALY (Disability-adjusted life years) lost, combined with death rates, gives a measure of overall population health – WHO.
Cf. disability, burden of disease, death rate, health, World Health Organization

Disappearance, forced disappearances The arrest, abduction, forced detention and cutting off communication of persons against their will, by or without the approval of the State or of a political organization, accompanied by refusal of the latter to acknowledge that abduction has taken place and denial of information on the fate of those abducted, thereby placing them outside the protection of the law. This is considered a crime against humanity. Example: disappearances in certain South American states during dictatorship.
Cf. crimes against humanity, human rights, deportation, man-conceived disaster

Disarmament The process and regulations concerning the reduction of a military establishment to levels defined by international agreement.
Cf. arms control

Disaster The result of a vast ecological breakdown in the physical and functional relations between man and his environment, caused by nature or man, a serious and sudden event (or slow, as in drought) on such a scale that available resources cannot meet the requirements, and the stricken community needs extraordinary efforts to cope with the damaging situation, often with outside help or international aid – Gunn.
Sn: catastrophe
Cf. natural disaster, man-made disaster, technological disaster, toxicological disaster, creeping disaster, fire disaster, environmental disaster, complex disaster, man-conceived disaster, humanitarian assistance

Disaster act (law) National legislation that provides the government or its appointed executive with special powers to mobilize the efforts and resources of the nation in face of a disaster or major emergency.
Cf. disaster legislation

Disaster assistance National or international aid, financial, technical or in-kind, to counter a particular or all phases of a disaster, from prevention and mitigation to immediate relief, reconstruction and rehabilitation.

Cf. technical assistance, technical cooperation, international assistance, humanitarian assistance, relief, disaster relief code of ethics

Disaster assessment/analysis Cf. assessment, disaster

Disaster convergence Cf. convergence in disasters

Disaster damage probability Cf. disaster damage formula

Disaster epidemiology The medical discipline, now extended to other fields, that studies the influence of such factors as lifestyle, biological constitution and other personal and social determinants on the incidence and distribution of disease, both under normal circumstances and in markedly changed disaster situations.
Cf. epidemiology, disaster medicine

Disaster fatigue A variety of emotional reactions and psychological problems and physical disorders can follow long-drawn emergency situations and disasters, including (a) under-reaction, confusion, stunned, unresponsive; (b) overreaction, unconnected hyperactivity; (c) deep grief with apathy, exhaustion, guilt; (d) physical disorders of diarrhoea, vomiting, immobility, limb paraesthesia and paralysis; (e) burn out; etc.

Disaster health Sn: disaster medicine

Disaster health diplomacy Negotiations, decisions and actions, usually undertaken under emergency conditions, based on long-term State and non-State preventive policies, alliances, available resources and organizational strategies with the view to ensuring the most effective response possible under adverse conditions.
Cf. humanitarian diplomacy, Surgeons OverSeas, global health diplomacy, disaster legislation, disaster medicine, disaster management

Disaster hospital capacity Cf. mass casualty situation

Disaster legislation The body of laws that govern and designate responsibility for disaster management in the nation concerning the various phases of disaster. Attempts are currently being made to introduce international disaster legislation.
Cf. disaster act (law)

Disaster management The study and collaborative application, by the various pertinent disciplines and governmental authorities, of decision-making processes, management techniques and resource utilization, to the entire process and different phases of a disaster, from prevention and preparedness to planning, immediate response, damage reduction, rehabilitation, reconstruction and development.
Cf. disaster mitigation, disaster preparedness, disaster team, disaster epidemiology, disaster probability, coping capacity, crisis, measures of effectiveness, plan, Utstein

Disaster medicine The study and collaborative application of various health disciplines – e.g. paediatrics, epidemiology, communicable diseases, nutrition, public health, emergency surgery, social medicine, military medicine, community care, international health – to the prevention, immediate response and rehabilitation of the health and humanitarian problems arising from disaster, in cooperation with other disciplines involved in comprehensive disaster management – Gunn.
Sn: disaster health

50

Cf. Centre for Research on the Epidemiology of Disasters (CRED), European Centre for Disaster Medicine (CEMEC), World Health Organization (WHO), humanitarian medicine, military medicine, International Association for Humanitarian Medicine (IAHM)

Disaster mitigation Separate and aggregate measures taken prior to or following a disaster to reduce the severity of human and material damage caused by it.
Cf. damage investigation, disaster management, disaster prevention

Disaster phases Cf. phases of disaster

Disaster preparedness The aggregate of measures to be taken in view of disasters, consisting of plans and action programmes designed to minimize loss of life and damage, to organize and facilitate effective rescue and relief and to rehabilitate after disaster. Preparedness requires the necessary legislation and means to cope with disaster or similar emergency situations. It is also concerned with forecasting and warning, the education and training of the public, organization and management, including plans, training of personnel, the stockpiling of supplies and ensuring the needed funds, personnel and other resources.
Cf. emergency, relief, supplies

Disaster prevention The aggregate of approaches and measures to ensure that human action or natural phenomena do not cause or result in disaster or similar emergency. It implies the formulation and implementation of long-range policies and programmes to eliminate or prevent the occurrence of disasters. Based on vulnerability analysis of risks, it also includes legislation and regulatory measures in the field of town planning, public works, environmental development and public awareness.

Disaster probability formula Cf. damage probability formula

Disaster reduction All decisions, actions, standards (preparedness, prevention), taken prior to relevant responses provided after a disaster, with the view to minimizing (mitigation) the damaging effects of a disaster.
Cf. disaster management, disaster preparedness, disaster prevention, disaster mitigation

Disaster Relief Code of Conduct A Code of Conduct introduced in 1994 by the Red Cross and several NGOs to establish self-regulation and standards in the provision of humanitarian aid. They stipulate that (1) the humanitarian imperative comes first, (2) aid is given without conditions and priorities are set on the basis of needs alone, (3) aid will not be used for political or religious purposes, (4) aid workers will not be instruments of government policy, (5) the culture and customs of the victims will be respected, (6) disaster workers will favour local capacities and UN participation, (7) programme beneficiaries will be included in relief management, (8) aid must meet basic needs and future vulnerabilities, (9) relief workers will stand accountable both to the aid recipients and to donors and (10) in all press and promotions, the dignity of the victims must be assured as human beings – G-IDNDR.
Cf. disaster assistance, Sphere Project, equity, custom, accountability

Disaster Research Center, Delaware Major academic and operational centre at the University of Delaware on all aspects of disaster. Important research and publications.

Disaster risk Cf. risk, risk management

Disaster severity scales
Disaster severity overall: de Boer (Cf.);
Disaster comparative magnitude: Bradford (Cf.);
Earthquake: intensity: Mercalli (Cf.); magnitude: Richter (Cf.);
European Macroseismic Scale (Cf.);
Hurricane: Beaufort (Cf.);
Nuclear bomb: Megaton (Cf.);
Nuclear reactor accident: INES: International Nuclear Event Scale (Cf.);
Sea state: Douglas (Cf.); Forel (Cf.);
Tornado: Fujita-Pearson (Cf.);
Wind force: Beaufort (Cf.)

Disaster severity score An attempt at scoring the severity of a disaster by attributing a figure, from 0 to 13, to the various parameters that characterize a disaster, such as the number of wounded, number of dead, the extent of the disaster, site, rescue time, severity of injuries, nature of the disaster, etc. – de Boer.

Disaster subculture Mechanisms, systems, adaptive attitudes and a way of life that certain communities living in known disaster areas, such as near floodlands, at the foot of a volcano or in the path of repeated tornadoes, develop as coping behaviour in response to the potential impact and "live with the hazard", Examples· Bangladesh, Carribbean, Mount Etna.
Cf. coping behaviour, adaptability

Disaster team Multidisciplinary, multisectoral group of persons qualified to evaluate a disaster and to bring the necessary relief.

Cf. disaster medicine, disaster prevention, emergency relief, international assistance

Disaster victim Person or population stricken directly or indirectly by a disaster.
Cf. disaster

Disastrology The science, practice and management of all types of major natural and man-made emergencies or disasters.
Sn: oxyology (rarely used)
Cf. disaster

Discrimination A person's, group's or government's negative view, intention and/or action based on the belief that a particular person, group or community is inferior, unworthy and undesirable due to a difference in race, religion, colour, nationality, conscience, political opinion, gender, facies, mental or physical handicap, socio-economic level or any imagined degradation. This is a violation of human rights.
Cf. human rights, Universal Declaration of Human Rights, xenophobia

Disease monitoring Sn: disease surveillance

Disease surveillance Health system used to monitor, observe and evaluate on a continuing basis the progress of a disease with the view to preventing or curing it.
Cf. disease monitoring, surveillance

Disease transmission Cf. transmission, communicable disease

Disinfectant Chemical substance used locally to destroy germs on the body or in the environment and to prevent their multiplication.
Cf. infection

Disinfection Destruction of germs or infectious agents outside the human body by chemical or physical means.

Cf. disinfectant, disinfestation

Disinfestation Technique or process used to destroy parasites, insects and other undesirable small animal species such as arthropods or rodents present on the person, on clothing, domestic animals or in the environment. Delousing is disinfestation against body lice.

Sn: disinsection

Cf. disinfection, fumigation, pesticide

Disinsection Cf. disinfestation

Displaced person(s) Persons who, for different reasons or circumstances – natural disasters, wars, conflicts or internal troubles – have been compelled to leave their homes. They may reside in their own country (internally displaced) or may not reside in their country of origin, but are not legally regarded as refugees.

Sn: DP

Cf. exodus, refugee, internally displaced person IDP

DNA/Deoxyribonucleic acid Abbreviation for deoxyribonucleic acid, present in chromosomes and carrier of genetic information. Used also for forensic identification of persons.

Cf. chromosome

Doha Declaration The health and trade Declaration on the TRIPS Agreement on public health made in Doha in 2001. Cf. TRIPS

Donation Material or monetary assistance extended without financial remuneration to a country, community or organization. Material, non-monetary assistance is called in-kind donation.

Cf. donor, donee

Donee Sn: beneficiary, recipient

Donor Disasters: A country, organization or agency that provides relief or, in different ways, comes to the assistance of a population in disaster.

Cf. aid, assistance, international assistance, technical assistance

Medicine: Blood donor, a person who agrees to the removal of a portion of his or her blood for transfusion to another person for therapeutic purposes.

Tissue donor: A person who agrees to give a portion of his or her body (other than blood or organ) to another person for therapeutic purposes, e.g. skin for burn treatment.

Organ donor: A person who agrees to the removal of an organ, e.g. kidney, for transplantation into another person for therapeutic purposes.

Donor agency Agency or organization that provides free emergency relief to a disaster stricken country or community without political or other considerations.

Cf. voluntary agency

Donor assessment Cf. humanitarian response index, good humanitarian donorship, DARA

Dose

1. In pharmacology, the strength or amount of medicament prescribed for each individual application.
2. In radioactivity, the amount of ionizing radiation absorbed by the exposed body.

   Cf. absorbed dose, collective dose, lethal dose, LD50, maximum acceptable dose, retained dose

Douglas scale Numerical scale from 0 to 9, indicating the state of the sea.

0 flat sea, 1 ripples, 2 calm sea, 3 small waves, 4 choppy, 5 waves and swells, 6 large waves and swells, 7 heavy sea, 8 very heavy sea, 9 huge swell.

Cf. Beaufort scale, swell, wave, Forel scale

Dracunculiasis A helminth infection transmitted by contaminated water.

Can cause a metre-long worm from a leg ulcer. A neglected tropical disease.
Sn: Guinea worm disease
Cf. neglected tropical diseases

Drainage Gradual evacuation of excess water from the more common surface run-off of wetlands (surface drainage) or from the ground (subsurface drainage) generally to improve agriculture.

Drainage basin Region drained by a part or the whole of one or several water channels.
Sn: catchment basin
Cf. catchment area, river basin, watershed

Dried full-cream milk Sn: dried whole milk

Dried skimmed milk Powdered food product processed by industrial drying and pulverization of skimmed milk. Such milk may lack some nutritional elements such as vitamin A.
Sn: DSM, skimmed milk powder
Cf. dried whole milk, vitamin A deficiency

Dried whole milk Powdered food product processed by industrial drying and pulverization of full-cream milk. Such milk may lack some nutritional elements.
Sn: dried full-cream milk, full-cream milk powder, DFCM, DWM
Cf. dried skimmed milk, food mixtures

Drift Any uncontrolled displacement of a floating or submerged object through the action of the wind or currents.

Drinking water Water that is agreeable to drink, does not present health hazards and whose quality is normally regulated by legislation. Essential to life.
Sn: potable water

Droit d'ingérence French term for the right to intervene. R2P

Drone A pilotless distance-guided military aircraft used for targeting and for reconnaissance.

Drowning An acute life-threatening event in which a person's nasal and pulmonary airways are suddenly obstructed by being submerged in liquid (usually water), leading to serious impairment of breathing, which calls for immediate disobstruction and life support to avert death.
Cf. ALS, waterboarding

Drought Climatic period with prolonged absence of rain during which time the degree of rainfall, expressed in millimetres, is less than twice the mean temperature, expressed in degrees Celsius, causing a shortage in needed water supply. Drought can be a disaster. (a) Agricultural drought is the lack of adequate soil moisture needed for certain crops to grow and thrive after a meteorological drought. (b) Meteorological drought is a deviation of the normal conditions of precipitation over a period of time in a specific region. (c) Hydrological drought occurs when precipitation has been reduced for an extended period of time, and water supplies in streams, lakes, rivers and reservoirs are deficient. (d) Socio-economic drought occurs when physical water supplies are so low that they negatively affect the social and economic conditions in the affected community.
UNCCD is the United Nations Convention to Combat Drought and Desertification.
Cf. aridity, desertification, disaster, precipitation, Sahel

Drug In its normal connotation, it means a therapeutic medicine and a pharmaceutical product, and usually druggists are pharmacists. But by deformed usage, drug has come to refer also to habit-forming, dependency-producing and often lethal, illegal substances.

The United Nations has established the UN Office for Drug Control and Crime Prevention.

Cf. narcotrafficking, mafia, dependence

Drug resistance The capacity acquired by microorganisms or parasites to survive, and eventually to multiply, in the presence of a medicament which would normally destroy them or prevent them from reproducing. By extension, drug-resistant disease. e.g. chloroquine-resistant malaria.

Cf. adaptation, habituation

Drugs for Neglected Diseases Initiative/DNDi DNDi is a non-profit product development endeavour that carries out research and development of new and better medicaments for neglected and rare diseases.

Cf. neglected diseases

Dry season In a tropical climate, period of the year characterized by very low or absence of rainfall.

Cf. drought, tropical climate

Dune A ridge or mound of sand or fine loose earth. Aeolian dunes are built up by the wind, hydraulic dunes by water currents.

Durban Declaration – Racism The World Conference Against Racism, Racial Discrimination, Xenophobia and Related Intolerance, held in 2001, South Africa, passed resolutions and decisions on these important issues.

Cf. racism, xenophobia, discrimination, human rights

Durra Black millet, grain of sorghum.

Dust bowl Ascending whirl of over-heated air carrying with it fine particles which subsequently remain suspended in the air.

Dust devil Sn: dust whirl

Dust whirl Aggregate of particles of dust or sand, sometimes accompanied by small litter raised from the ground, in the form of a whirling column of varying height with a small diameter and almost vertical axis.

Sn: dust devil, sand whirl

Dwelling Any covered and sheltered space, such as a house, hut or tent, reserved to provide living quarters for one or more households.

Dyke A construction along a coast or river bank for the protection of people, port facilities or of water reservoirs.

Cf. levee

Dynamic testing Actual experimental testing and analysis of the response of structures subjected to simulated natural and varied other stresses.

Dysentery
1. A general term used for different kinds of unspecified diarrhoea or gastroenteritis.
2. Specific infection of the colon, such as shigellosis (bacillary dysentery) or amoebiasis (amoebic dysentery).

   Cf. diarrhoeal diseases, enteric diseases, infection

Dyspnoea A respiratory symptom that may indicate shortness of breath, or breathlessness, tightness in the chest, feeling of suffocation, pain on breathing or feeling of not getting enough air.

Cf. asphyxia, respiratory distress

E

Early warning Timely, understandable and useful information given to the population and institutions concerning a probable oncoming disaster, based on knowledgeable information and authoritative decisions, with the view to taking appropriate shelter, effective   actions   and   relevant

responses in order to minimize the expected damage.
Cf. alarm

Early warning system The set of capacities needed to generate and disseminate timely and meaningful warning information to enable individuals, communities and organizations threatened by a hazard to prepare and to act appropriately and in sufficient time to reduce the possibility of harm or loss – UNISDR.
A warning system comprises knowledge of the risks, monitoring and forecasting of the hazards, dissemination of the alerts and local capacities to respond to the warning.
Cf. alert, warning

Earth flow Mass of water-logged earth, sliding by gravity along a slope at a relatively slow speed of a few kilometres per hour.
Sn: mudslide

Earth station Communications station situated either on land (or ship or on an airplane), with the purpose of communicating with one or several stations and linked with other earth stations through a space network.
Cf. geostatic station

Earth Summit, Rio United Nations conference held in Rio de Janeiro in 1992 that established the principle and need of sustainable development.

Earthquake The violent shaking of the ground produced by deep seismic waves, beneath the epicentre, generated by a sudden decrease or release in a volume of rock of elastic strain accumulated over a long time in regions of seismic activity (tectonic earthquake). The magnitude of an earthquake is represented by the Richter scale, the intensity by the Mercalli scale.
Cf. epicentre, Mercalli scale, Richter scale, European macroseismic scale,

seismic sea wave, seismic sounding, seismograph, seismoscope, quake, tsunami

Earthquake scales Cf. Richter scale, Mercalli scale, European macroseismic scale

Earthquake swarm A series of minor seismic shocks limited in time and space but which cannot be identified as a principal shock.

Eating unit A group of persons gathered together and sharing food prepared by the same kitchen or in several communal kitchens.

Ebb Receding movement of the sea water or reflux of the tide.
Sn: recession

Ebola fever Very serious and highly contagious disease caused by the very virulent Ebola virus. Closely related to the Marburg virus.
Sn: African haemorrhagic fever

Echinococcosis Sn: hydatid disease
Cf. neglected tropical disease

ECHO Acronym for European Community Humanitarian Office. A major source of humanitarian aid, the European Union provides emergency relief to victims of both natural and man-made disasters and helps in preparedness and prevention projects, not limited to Europe.
Cf. European Union, OCHA

Ecology The science that studies the relationships of living organisms between themselves and with their environment.

Economic development Increase in monetary terms in the national product of a country and in the resultant material and social well-being and individual income of its population.
Cf. development, country economic categories, sustainable development, MDGs

Economic refugee(s) Persons or groups of people who decide to migrate internally or leave for another country because of poverty, low incomes or difficulty in subsistence and in the hope of better incomes and improved quality of life. Juridically, they are not recognized as refugees.
Cf. environmental refugee, refugee

Economy class syndrome Deep vein thrombosis of the lower legs and/or pulmonary embolism (which can be fatal) that develops in air passengers in crammed (economy class) conditions during or following a long flight.
Has also been observed among disaster victims crammed for long periods in crowded shelters, without exercise – Ukai.

Ecosystem Contraction for ecological system. Basic ecological unit formed by the biotope (living environment) and the animal and vegetable organisms naturally living there and interacting as a single functional entity.
Cf. ecology, environment

Ecotoxicology Study of the effects and potential adverse events caused by chemical agents on the environment and on the general ecosystem, including – but not necessarily – on human health – after WHO.
Cf. ecosystem, ecology

Effective life/radionuclide The time needed for the quantity of a given radionuclide to be reduced by half, either through loss of radioactivity or by biological elimination.
Cf. half-life, radioactivity

Effectiveness Measure of the extent to which planned activities are realized and planned results obtained – ISO 9000 (2000).
Cf. efficient

Efficient A health plan or action is efficient if the effort expended on it is as good as possible in relation to the resources devoted to it. – HFA

Effluent Residual waters, treated or not, of agricultural, industrial or urban provenance.

e-Health A system of electronic management of health information and services. (Not to be confused with mHealth.)
Cf. mHealth

El Niño A climatic phenomenon of the southern oceans with global and long-term meteorological and agricultural repercussions. It occurs every 2–7 years in an 18-month sequence of events extending across the entire Pacific and Indian Oceans. It begins with an anomalous warming of the upper part of the ocean off the west coast of South America, which can lead to drought, monsoon failure and disastrous winds in areas as scattered as Indonesia, the Amazon valley, Australia or Melanesia. The opposite phenomena are referred to as La Niña. In recent years, with climate change, the pattern is showing unusual changes.
Cf. global warming

Electrical burn Burn damage to the tissues by passage of an electric current which is converted into thermal energy. This energy is proportional to the square of the current intensity in amperes and to the resistance of the conductor in ohms. The effects caused by electric energy depend on the type of circuit, voltage and amperage of current, resistance, route of the current and duration of contact. Electrocution is a most severe electrical burn with the strong current passing through the body, often causing death.
Cf. burns, electrocution

Electrocution Cf. electrical burn

Electromagnetic pulse The very brief and intense pulse of electromagnetic radiation emitted following a high-altitude nuclear explosion, causing extensive interference over a vast area at ground level, resulting in neutralization of telecommunications, radio broadcasts, electronic controls, electrotechnical equipment, hospitals, transport or at home.

Sn: EMP

Electron The elementary particle of negative charge in all atoms.

Cf. ionizing radiation, proton

Elements at risk The population, buildings and civil engineering works, economic activities, public services and infrastructure, etc., at risk in a given area – UN.

Cf. risk, risk indicator, risk map, specific risk

eLENA e-Library of Evidence for Nutrition Actions (WHO). Strives to clarify electronically the vast and often conflicting evidence, information and advice that exist on effective, preventive and therapeutic nutrition interventions.

Emaciation The exhaustion of essential cellular elements, mainly in muscle and adipose tissue, following privation of food and often associated with infections and debilitating illnesses.

Embargo An order forbidding certain activities, often accompanied with certain penalties or sanctions in case of non-compliance. Article 41, Chapter VII of the UN charter provides for embargoes on a country that may pose a threat to peace, a breakdown of peace or an act of aggression, e.g. Iraq against Kuwait. Usually goods considered humanitarian, such as food and medicine, may be exempted.

In journalism, an embargo is a request not to publish a certain declaration or news item before a specified date.

Emergency A sudden and usually unforeseen event that must be countered immediately to minimize the consequences. If the event is major, the term disaster is often used. With rational planning, emergencies can be tackled with less "surprise" and more effectively.

Emergency Events Database EM-DAT, a compilation created by CRED that gives direct access statistics through its website. Has information on natural disasters from 1990 onwards.

Cf. CE-DAT, Centre for Research in Epidemiology of Disasters

Emergency feeding Distribution of food to communities, families and individuals who are cut off from their normal food supplies or are unable to prepare their own food as a result of a natural or man-made disaster such as famine, flood, earthquake, war.

Cf. famine, food, food relief, relief, supplies

Emergency health kit Basic drugs and medical equipment calculated for the emergency needs of a population of 10,000 persons over three months. One pre-packaged kit contains 10 identical smaller kits, each for 1,000 persons.

Sn: WHO Emergency Health Kit (the previous name)

Cf. stockpile, supplies, World Health Organization

Emergency life support Urgent measures taken to keep a critically ill patient alive, usually in a hospital critical care unit.

Cf. basic life support, advanced life support, cardiopulmonary-cerebral resuscitation, survival chain

Emergency management The organization and management of all resources and responsibilities for addressing all aspects of emergencies, in particular preparedness, response and initial recovery – UNISDR.

Emergency medical services The system of various resources, organization, facilities and personnel necessary to deliver the needed medical care to those with an unpredicted immediate need outside a hospital and continued care once in an established emergency facility.
Sn: EMS
Cf. first aid, life support, oxyology, prehospital medicine

Emergency Risk Management and Humanitarian Response/WHO ERM, department at WHO for emergency humanitarian management, now expanded to include Health Action in Crises (HAC), Polio Eradication and Country Collaboration (PEC) clusters.

Emergency relief
1. Urgent aid given to relieve suffering and hardship arising from a sudden or unexpected event.
2. Immediate assistance given to persons who are deprived of the essential needs of life following a natural or man-induced disaster.
Cf. disaster, relief

Emergent country An imprecise term denoting a developing country that is relatively advanced (or advancing) towards becoming a full-fledged developed or industrial country as measured by its economic progress.
Cf. country economic category, BRICS

Emigrant Person who moves to another country for personal, economic, social or political reasons. Distinguish from migrant, immigrant and refugee.
Cf. immigrant, migrant, refugee

Emigration The act of leaving one's country or place of residence with the intention of settling in another country or place. Emigration from a country does not imply the loss of nationality of that country, and it does not confer refugee status.
Cf. exodus, immigration, migration

Empowerment Enablement by education or by law, giving authority where it was previously lacking. In medicine, it means facilitating and recognizing in persons or patients their right and ability to control their own health problems and health-care decisions.
Cf. ethics in health

Encephalitis Serious neurological disease caused by inflammation of the brain elements due to viral, microbial or parasitic infection.
Cf. cerebrospinal meningitis, bovine spongiform encephalopathy

Endemic disease The usual presence or prevalence of a disease in a given geographical area. Hyperendemic expresses a persistence in excess of expected endemicity. Pandemic is the presence of a disease, at the same time, in important proportions, throughout the world. Example: AIDS.
Cf. endemicity, epidemic, pandemic

Endemic treponematoses A group of chronic bacterial infections – yaws, pinta, endemic syphilis (bijel) – caused by treponemes that mainly affect the skin.
Cf. neglected tropical diseases

Endemic(ity) Habitual presence or recurrence of a disease, e.g. cholera, or other phenomena, e.g. cyclones, in a given population or region. Example: both are endemic in the Bay of Bengal area.
Cf. endemic disease

Energy assessment Comparative study of the sum of calories provided by food and of their utilization for such biological requirements as tissue maintenance and growth. Assessment can be established for an organism, an individual or a population.
Cf. energy requirements

Energy requirements Quantity of energy required to maintain the weight equilibrium of an average individual of given sex and age in good health.
Cf. energy assessment, health, needs.

Energy problem The impact of the aggregate patterns and extents of energy consumption upon the environment and the capacity of that environment and society to meet the energy needs for an equitable and sustainable development.

Enriched food Sn: fortified food

Enriched uranium Sn: U308
Cf. uranium

Enteral Medication given via the alimentary tract, by mouth or by rectal introduction. Not by injection.

Enteric diseases A general term for a variety of infectious intestinal diseases due to a number of known causes (amoebae, intestinal parasites, worms, bacilli, vibrio cholerae) or unknown causes transmitted through various mechanisms (food, water, direct contact). Can be of sudden diarrhoeal onset, chronic or in carrier state, all with danger of transmission. Disaster conditions facilitate and aggravate the disease with risk of epidemics, especially among children.
Cf. amoebiasis, cholera, diarrhoeal diseases, dysentery, oral rehydration, typhoid

Environment The aggregate, at any given time, of the physical, chemical and biological agents and social factors that can have a direct or indirect, immediate or late effect on living organisms and on human activities.

Environmental change Modification, favourable or unfavourable, of the ecological state and environment.
Cf. ecology, environment, environmental impact assessment

Environmental degradation Cf. environmental pollution

Environmental disruption Any physical, chemical and/or biological changes in the ecosystem – or the resource base – that render it temporarily or permanently unsuitable to support human life – UNEP. Such deterioration is a cause of environmental refugees.
Sn: environmental impact
Cf. environment, environmental refugees, refugee

Environmental health The science and measures that aim at creating the environmental conditions most conducive to health.
Cf. environmental hygiene, public health, sanitary engineering

Environmental hygiene The measures that aim at creating favourable environmental conditions for health and disease prevention.
Cf. environmental health, environmental pollution, public health

Environmental impact Cf. environmental change

Environmental impact assessment Investigation of the eventual positive or negative effect of any new factor on a given environment and its ecological equilibrium.
Sn: EIA
Cf. environmental change

Environmental pollution Unfavourable changes and degradation of one or more aspects or elements of the environment by noxious biological, industrial, chemical or radioactive wastes, from debris of man-made, especially non-biodegradable products and from mismanagement and inconsiderate use of ecological resources.

Sn: environmental degradation

Cf. air pollution, atmospheric pollution, environment, environmental disruption, environmental refugee, man-made disaster, oil pollution, oil slick

Environmental refugees(s) People who have been forced to leave their original habitat, temporarily or permanently, because of marked disruption of the environment through natural or man-made causes that jeopardized their existence and/or seriously affected the quality of their lives – UNEP.

There are broadly three categories of environmental refugees: (1) people who have been temporarily displaced because of environmental stress and who return when the disruption is over, (2) people who become permanently displaced and must resettle in a new area because of permanent changes in their original habitat, such as the establishment of huge dams and (3) individuals or groups of people who emigrate internally or abroad, temporarily or permanently, in search of a better quality of life, e.g. leaving a drought-hit area for more fertile land.

Cf. environment, environmental disruption, refugee, economic refugee

Environmental sustainability index A scale from 0 to 100 that rates the environmental performance of a country or region, based on the total scores of about 60 variables covering the following five categories: (a) human vulnerability to environment, e.g. disease and available potable water, (b) social institutional capacity, e.g.

to respond to or promote environmental issues, (c) societal stresses on the environment, e.g. pollution, urbanization, (d) global conscience, e.g. the community's efforts to diminish global warming, and (e) level of environmental facilities, e.g. water quality systems.

Sn: ESI

Cf. environment, sustainable development

Epidemic
1. An unusual increase in the number of cases of an infectious or parasitic disease which already exists in an endemic state in the region or population concerned.
2. The appearance of a more or less important number of cases of an infectious disease introduced in a region or population that is usually free from that disease.

Cf. communicable disease, endemic, pandemic, infectious disease, potential epidemic, threatened epidemic

Epidemic/pandemic alerts Cf. WHO epidemic alert degrees, potential epidemic, threatened epidemic

Epidemiology The medical discipline that studies the influence of such factors as the lifestyle, biological constitution and other personal or social determinants on the incidence and distribution of disease.

Cf. disaster medicine, disaster epidemiology

Epizootic disease Affecting simultaneously many animals of the same kind in the same region and rapidly spreading. Also refers to an extensive outbreak of an epizootic disease. Examples: mad cow disease, rabies. The World Organization for Animal Health (OIE – Organisation Internationale des Epizooties) is concerned with these problems.

Cf. bovine spongiform encephalopathy, BSE, mad cow disease, zoonosis, OIE

Equal access The social and legislative mechanisms that provide equal opportunity of obtaining available care and services for equal needs, based on a study of such needs, with a fair distribution throughout the country for easily reachable access without social, financial or other barriers.
Cf. access, equity

Equatorial climate Climate characterized by a twin season of rain during May–June and October–November, with a short dry season towards the month of August (in the northern hemisphere).
Cf. dry season, rainy season

Equatorial depression Zone of relatively low pressure situated between the subtropical anticyclones of the two hemispheres.
Cf. anticyclone, atmospheric depression, depression

Equity in health The policy and practices that provide everyone, without distinction, a fair opportunity to equal access to available care for equal need, equal utilization for equal need and equal quality care for all – (after WHO).
Cf. humanitarian medicine, ethics, World Health Organization

Erosion The degradation and transformation of the soil and of the earth's crust due to the action of water, wind and other atmospheric agents.
Cf. anthropic erosion, continental erosion, wind erosion

Eruption The sudden surfacing of solid and gaseous material from the depths of the earth.
Cf. volcano

Essential bodily needs The normal body has certain physiological needs for which minimum health standards have been established and which must be provided even under the most difficult circumstances, e.g. in wars, refugee camps, disaster situations
Cf. water, shelter, sanitation, space requirements

Essential medicines The WHO model list of essential medicines. Contains a core of 325 medicaments for the minimum needs of basic health care, listing the most efficacious, safe and cost-effective medicines for priority conditions. A complementary list presents essential medicines for priority diseases for which specialized diagnostic and/or investigative facilities and/or specialist training are required.
A separate list of essential medicines and equipment for disaster situations is the WHO Emergency Health Kit. (Cf.)

Essential surgery Surgical investigations and procedures that can be carried out in rural or district first referral or remote hospitals, mainly in developing and poorer countries with less advanced facilities, by low-level paramedical and nursing staff trained for such events or by doctors experienced to work under such shortages. The facility strengthens primary healthcare services for injuries, pregnancy-related complications, fractures, debilitating hernias, abscesses and other essential or life-saving interventions.
IFSC/SCES.
Cf. GIEESC, surgical conditions humanitarian surgery

The Ethical Globalization Initiative
Cf. Realizing Rights

Ethics Relating to morals, treating of moral principles, rules of personal and societal conduct, respect for the person, equitable, humane and fair action.
Cf. disaster relief code of ethics, ethics in health care

Ethics in health care In the practice and administration of health care, covers (a) moral principles of behaviour, (b) professional standards guiding and expected of all involved in health care, (c) patient respect and empowerment and (d) abidance by therapeutic deontological precepts.
Cf. empowerment, humanitarian medicine, equity in health

Ethnic cleansing New term for an age-old and decidedly unclean policy of some totalitarian governments aiming at removing through hatred, intimidation, deportation, killing, genocide or any other form of force, certain groups or minorities within the country in order to homogenize the national population, acquire land, pamper to extremist pride and ensure control.
Cf. deportation, disappearances, discrimination, ethnic group, minorities, Universal Declaration of Human Rights, man-conceived disaster, genocide

Ethnic group/population An organic group of individuals sharing distinctive common traits, customs, language and culture that distinguishes them from others in the same or different country. The term sometimes refers to such groups as a minority in a larger population.

EU 501/82 Rules European Union Regulations and emergency plans for any industrial activity that may be "a major accident hazard".
Cf. Seveso, toxicological disaster

Euro The currency unit of the European Union.
The Regional Office for Europe of the World Health Organization.

Europe-Third World Centre Cf. Centre Europe-Tiers Monde/Université de Lausanne

Euro-Mediterranean Council for Burns and Fire Disaster Expanded activity and new name of the Mediterranean Council for Burns and Fire Disasters (Cf.)

European Centre for Disaster Medicine/CEMEC Intergovernmental centre established in San Marino under the aegis of the Council of Europe, to promote prevention and mitigation of the effects of natural and technological disasters through research, training programmes and international collaboration, in particular among European countries. Known under its Italian acronym, CEMEC.
Cf. Council of Europe, disaster medicine

European Commission The executive arm of the European Union. (Do not confuse with the Council of Europe.)
Cf. European Union

European Commission Humanitarian Operations Commonly known as ECHO, the important disaster prevention and emergency response system of the European Union, very active and not limited to Europe.

European Convention on Human Rights Established by the Council of Europe, a fundamental international instrument that defines in 18 articles the inalienable rights and freedoms of every person everywhere. The European Court of Human Rights ensures the observance of these engagements.
Cf. Council of Europe, human rights, Universal Declaration of Human Rights

European Humanitarian Personnel Network In response to the recurrent difficulty of recruiting trained health personnel in emergency situations and for disaster response, this network tries to recruit, train and maintain a registry of relevant health personnel for emergency humanitarian work.

Cf. EURO, EU, JICA

European Macroseismic Scale (EMS-12) A summary and simplified scale of the Council of Europe with 12° of earthquake intensity:

Intensity I: not felt, II: scarcely felt, III: weak, IV: largely observed, V: strong, VI: slight damage, VII: damage, VIII: heavy damage, IX: destruction, X: heavy destruction, XI: devastation, XII: complete devastation. – G.IDNDR

Sn: EMS-12

Cf. Richter scale, Mercally scale

European Union/EU The institutional arrangements bringing together the European Communities, with open borders (Schengen accord) and a common currency (Euro), with the ultimate goal of gradually integrating their economies and moving towards political unity. It is currently comprised of 27 European states. Formerly known as the Commission of European Communities or Common Market, the EU includes the European Parliament, the European Commission, the European Court of Justice, Europol and other instruments, in Brussels. The European Commission is EU's executive arm.

Major role in disaster prevention and response (ECHO). Do not confuse with Council of Europe.

Cf. Council of Europe, United Nations,

Euthanasia Allowing the death of a terminally or hopelessly sick or injured person (passive euthanasia) or causing the death of such a suffering person as an act of mercy (active euthanasia).

Evacuation An operation to clear a region of its inhabitants, generally under threat (e.g. conflict) or following a disaster.

Cf. disaster, evacuee, prevention

Evacuee A person temporarily displaced from one place to another, within the same area or another country, to safeguard his health and security.

Cf. evacuation, displaced person

Evaluation The process of determining the worth or significance of an activity or programme; an assessment as systematic and objective as possible, of a planned, ongoing or completed intervention – OECD.

Evaluation of disaster Detailed post-impact assessment of the disaster situation taking into account all aspects of the damage, including the physical site, built structures, disrupted social system, remaining health facilities, shelter, water supplies, food availability, mortality, communications, transport, disposal of the dead. Evaluation also points to the remaining needs and facilities for immediate reconstruction.

Evidence-based medicine The practice of medicine and the assessment of its efficacy based on criteria of preventive, diagnostic, therapeutic and comparative methods of scientifically proven evidence, with the goal of providing the best possible management of health and disease in the patient.

Excision (in genital mutilation) In female genital mutilation, the practice of ablating the prepuce and hood of the clitoris and the labia minora.

Sn: clitoridectomy

Cf. female genital mutilation, infibulation, introcision

Exodus The massive displacement of a population for various reasons, usually due to political and social conflict, civil or military strife, persecutions and other violations of human rights.
Cf. displaced persons, emigration, refugee, diaspora

Expanded Programme on Immunization The continuing programme of WHO for the systematic vaccination of all children against the following six diseases: diphtheria, pertussis, tetanus (DPT vaccine), poliomyelitis (P), tuberculosis (BCG vaccine) and measles.
Sn: EPI
Cf. immunization, vaccination, diphtheria, measles, poliomyelitis, tetanus, tuberculosis, whooping cough

Expatriate A national of a country who lives in another country and abides by the laws of the host country.
Sn: expat (colloquial)

Expert A qualified and experienced agent who, in his special field of competence, carries out operational, advisory, training or managerial tasks for or within a government or institution with the view to assisting in development or other national activity, such as disaster management.
Cf. delegate, technical assistance, representative

Explosivity index In volcanology, the percentage of pyroclastic ejecta within the total eruption product.
Cf. volcanic eruption, pyroclastic flow

Exponential growth Growth that is a simple function of the size of the growing subject, such that the larger the population, the faster its growth.
Cf. arithmetic growth

Exposure Radiation The radioactive contamination of a living or inanimate object by accident or design.

Environment: The long and damaging contact of a living being with the harsh elements of the environment, such as extremely cold weather.
Pollution: The undesirable contact of living and inanimate objects with pollutants in the atmosphere.
Fire: Structures that are at risk of catching fire by extension from a fire in the vicinity.

Extermination Intentional infliction of unacceptable conditions of life, inter alia deprivation of food, medicines, etc., calculated to bring about the destruction of part of a population – ICC.
Cf. genocide, International Criminal Court

Eye (of the storm) The calm central zone of low pressure (eye) of a cyclone. The violent wind circulation around it gyrates counterclockwise in the northern hemisphere and clockwise in the southern.
Cf. cyclone, hurricane, tropical cyclone, typhoon

Exxon Valdez On 24 March 1989, a huge oil tanker called Exxon Valdez ran aground at Prince William Sound, Alaska, spilling 38,000 tons of crude oil, affecting 1,200 miles of coastline, with extensive marine ecological damage and wiping out some 20 communities, though no human life was lost. Very serious technological, social, environmental and financial disaster.
Cf. oil spill, Bhopal, Chernobyl

F

Façade democracy A tendency to add qualifying adjectives and epithets to the concept of democracy, such as disciplined democracy, guided democracy, protected democracy,

etc., when the essential elements are missing and in effect diminishing the value of democracy.
Cf. democracy

Facies Appearance, of usually facial aspects, that may be associated with racial origin, creating unjust negative interpretations, bias and discrimination.
Cf. discrimination, racism

Failure The diminution or end of the capacity of a structure, item or system to perform its required function.
Cf. reliability

Falciparum malaria Malaria due to *Plasmodium falciparum*, the most dangerous form of malaria in children.
Cf. malaria

Fall Water – in liquid or solid state – precipitated from the atmosphere onto the ground.
Sn: precipitation

Falling cloud Volcanic cloud composed of the same elements as in glowing cloud, but projected almost vertically and falling back to earth. Example: the St. Vincent eruption of 1902.
Cf. glowing cloud, ash fall

Fallout In radioactivity: The deposition of radioactive materials in the atmosphere and on the earth. Such radioactivity in the atmosphere may arise from natural causes, from nuclear bomb explosions or from atomic reactor accidents inducing radioactivity and fission products.
Nuclear cloud is the deposition of nuclear material in the atmosphere, where it may move according to the winds or may be precipitated to earth with rain.
Global fallout is the deposition on the ground of radioactivity from a nuclear weapon exploded in the stratosphere.

Intermediate fallout is the deposition on the ground of radioactivity from a nuclear weapon exploded in the troposphere.
Local fallout is the deposition of radioactivity from a nuclear weapon, downwind at ground level, during the first 24 h after explosion on the ground.
Sn: radioactive fallout
Cf. ionizing radiation, nuclear war, nuclear winter, environmental refugee
In general: The unplanned and usually unexpected secondary effects of some human action. Example: overgrazing creating food shortage that causes population displacement.

Family (household) unit A dwelling inhabited by one household and providing the family atmosphere.
Sn: household unit Cf. dwelling, household

Family planning A way of thinking and living adopted voluntarily, on the basis of knowledge, attitudes and responsible decisions, by individuals and couples, in order to promote the health and welfare of the family group and thus contribute effectively to the social development of a country – WHO, 1975.
Cf. UNFPA

Famine A disastrous shortage of food affecting large numbers of people. It may be due to poor harvests following drought, floods, earthquake, war, social conflict, etc. A slow-onset disaster.
Cf. drought, food, food shortage, hunger, famine management

Famine management The aggregate of studies, information, planning and action to foresee, prevent, alleviate and manage a famine disaster. The joint WHO-CRED project of Consolidated Information System for Famine Management in Africa is a useful approach to such management.

Far-field In a nuclear incident, designates the area away from the immediately involved ground or zero zone ("near-field") and considered less dangerous but still bearing the contamination and damaging effects of the accident.
Cf. near-field, nuclear accident, ground zero, zone zero

FARC Hispano-American acronym for Fuerzas Armadas Revolucionarias de Colombia, the anti-government rebel political movement that controls a part of Colombia and is an important illicit base of coca production and cocaine trafficking that constitute a regional security problem.
Cf. drug trafficking, UN Office on Drugs and Crime

Fatality The severity of a disease as judged by the frequency of the deaths that occur among the patients of that disease in relation to the total number of sick persons. This concept is commonly employed to calculate the ratio of the number of fatal cases in a specific clinical or epidemiological experience. The ratio is disease specific: Thus, fatality in diphtheria is about 5%.
Sn: mortality
Cf. case fatality rate

Fatwa Arabic term for a formal Islamic religious legal opinion.
Cf. sharia

Fault (geological) In geology and seismology, the planar or gently curving fracture in the earth's crust across which displacement and sliding occur.
Cf. sliding fault, transform fault, fracture zone

Favela A disorganized collection of disorderly, unsanitary, paupers' dwellings.
Cf. shanty town (South American), slum

Fédération Dentaire Internationale/ World Dental Federation/FDI The world's major federation of national dental associations that promotes better oral health as a basic part of general health. Dental records are a fundamental element in forensic science and disaster medicine for identifying persons.

Female circumcision A euphemistic term for female genital mutilation.
Cf. female genital mutilation

Female genital mutilation Cruel and medically unnecessary modification of the female genitalia, practised in certain countries, especially in Africa, under the guise of cultural, religious or traditional obligation. May include incision/excision of the labia, clitoris, infibulectomy and other mutilations. Also called female circumcision. Condemned by WHO, the UN and women's organizations.
Cf. excision, infibulation, introcision

Filariasis A group of diseases in tropical and subtropical countries due to filarial worms and transmitted by mosquitoes and flies. Bancroftian filariasis may produce elephantiasis of the limbs, causing invalidity.
Cf. parasitic diseases

Fireball The tremendously hot and brilliant sphere of burning gases immediately following a nuclear explosion in the air.
Cf. conflagration, firestorm, superfire, nuclear warFirebreak
A natural or constructed discontinuity in a fuel bed utilized to segregate, stop and control the spread of fire or to provide a control line from which to suppress a fire – FAO.
Cf. barrier

Firebug Popular term for pyromaniac, an arsonist. Psychologically unstable and abnormal person with compulsive desire to set a fire and taking pathological pleasure out of it.

Cf. arson, forest fire

Fireproof The quality of a structure or object to resist fire either by its own nature or imparted to it by treatment with retardants so as to reduce the danger of fire starting or spreading.

Fire resistant The quality of a material or device to maintain its properties and function against exposure to fire under certain conditions.

Cf. fireproof, flameproof, fire retardant

Fire retardant Any physical or chemical substance – other than water – that is used to slow down or reduce a fire or flammability of a fuel.

Sn: retardant

Cf. fireproof, flameproof

Firestorm The coalescing of many fires into a single big fire creating a convective column, with very high temperatures. Firestorms and superfires are now believed to be the cause of the greatest number of casualties following nuclear war.

Cf. conflagration, fireball, superfire

Fire foam A physico-chemical extinguishing foamy material that, when applied to the flaming object or sea surface, blankets and adheres to the fuel, reducing the combustion.

Fire hazard A fuel source, identified by its nature, type, locality and accessibility, that determines the ease with which it can catch fire or the difficulty with which it can be put out.

Cf. fire, fireproof, forest fire, class of fire

Fire, natural Any fire started by natural causes, such as lightning, spontaneous combustion or volcanic activity. Thus, lightning fire, spontaneous fire, volcanic fire.

Cf. forest fire

Fire, Wildland Sn: Wildfire

First aid Immediate and temporary simple care given to the victim on the site of an accident or sudden sickness in order to stop bleeding, lessen pain, diminish suffering, avert complications and comfort the person until competent help or a physician is obtained.

Cf. Emergency Medical Services, prehospital medicine, rescue

First strike A pre-emptive attack using nuclear weapons.

Cf. nuclear war

Fissile Refers (1) to a nuclide capable of undergoing fission by interaction with slow neutrons. (2) Material containing one or more fissile nuclides – ISO.

Fission bomb Nuclear weapon in which the explosive power is derived from the fission of atomic nuclei, with liberation of energy and radiation. It is the basic nuclear weapon, popularly referred to as the atomic bomb. The bombs on Hiroshima and Nagasaki were fission bombs.

Sn: atom bomb

Cf. atomic bomb, fusion bomb, nuclear energy, nuclear war, kiloton

Fission (nuclear) The splitting (fission) of a heavy nucleus into two parts, with release of energy and neutrons.

Cf. fission bomb, fusion bomb, nuclear war, reactor

Fission-fusion-fission (F-F-F) bomb A nuclear weapon with energy release in three stages: (1) fission, acting as the trigger; (2) fusion, occurring at the high temperature created in the first stage; and (3) fission, by the neutrons emitted at fusion, in a uranium tamper – Rotblat.

Flameproof The property of a material or assemblage not to burst in flames during a lapse of time in a fire. Flame is ignited gas.

Cf. fireproof, fire resistant, retardant

Flammable/Flammability The characteristic and degree of ease with which any material will burn.
Sn: inflammable (attention, in UK English, flammable and inflammable are synonymous. As the latter – inflammable – may erroneously give the idea of non-flammable, it is safer to use the US term flammable rather than inflammable.)

Flash flood A local flood of sudden rise and short duration with great volume that causes inundation, generally due to very heavy rainfall in the vicinity.
Cf. precipitations, swell

Floating barrier A portable, inflatable device placed as an emergency on the surface of a water mass where oil spill has occurred, with the aim of controlling and barring the spread and aspirating the oil to limit further environmental pollution.
Sn: floating barrage, isolator, oil boom
Cf. environmental pollution, oil slick

Flood Overflow of areas which are not normally submerged, with water or stream that has broken its normal confines, and/or accumulated due to lack of drainage.

Flood control The management of water resources and prevention of accidents through construction of reservoirs, dams, embankments, diversion channels, etc., to avoid floods.

Flood tide Sn: rising tide

Floodplain An area adjacent to a river, formed by the repeated overflow of the natural channel bed – OFDA.
Cf. flood, precipitations, zoning

Floodway A bypass channel built from an upstream point in order to divert the flooding waters downstream in a controlled way.

Fluoridation Addition of certain prescribed quantities of fluoride to drinking water as a preventive measure against dental caries.

Focal depth In seismology, the vertical distance from the surface of the earth to the focus or point of origin of an earthquake.
Cf. earthquake, focus, ground zero

Focus In seismology, the point beneath the surface of the earth where an earthquake rupture originates – hypocentre – and from where seismic waves radiate.
Cf. earthquake, focal depth, hypocentre

Food Edible substance containing nutrients which, on ingestion, maintain the vital functions of a person or other living organism.
Cf. conventional food, fortified food, protective food, staple food

Food additive Substance intentionally added to food, generally in small quantities, to improve its physical or chemical properties (appearance, aroma, consistency, flavour) or preservation capacity, but not its nutritional value. Examples: colourant, emulsifier, stabilizer.
Cf. fortified food

Food aid Assistance rendered on an organized basis, free or on concessional terms, to provide food to a population group, community or country suffering from food shortage or insufficient development.
Cf. food relief, supplementary feeding programme

Food and Agriculture Organization/ FAO The UN specialized agency that aims to raise the levels of nutrition, to improve the production and distribution of all agricultural and food products from farms, forests and

fisheries and to eliminate hunger. It promotes improved soil and water management, better crop yields, healthier livestock and sound agricultural investment. Has an Office of Special Relief Operations (OSRO) for disaster situations and mobilizing resources. Coordinates with the World Food Programme (WFP).
Sn: FAO
Cf. drought, rural development, United Nations, World Food Programme

Food and nutrition indicators Quantified data that indicate the quantity and quality of foodstuffs available to a population. Examples: calories or proteins available per person and the need/availability ratio of a foodstuff.
Cf. nutritional state indicators, needs

Food availability indicators Cf. food and nutrition indicators

Food chain The sequence of transfer of matter and energy in the form of eatable material from organism to organism in ascending or descending trophic levels – WHO.

Food consumption survey Survey designed to elicit qualitative and quantitative information on food consumption in a given community or country.

Food enrichment Sn: food fortification
Cf. fortified food

Food fortification Food fortification and food enrichment are used interchangeably or synonymously.
Cf. fortified food

Food habits The ways in which an individual or group utilizes foods and consumes them in response to physiological, psychological, cultural, social and geographic influences.

Food hygiene That part of the science of hygiene that deals with the principles and methods of sanitation applied to the quality of foodstuffs, to their processing, preparation, conservation and consumption by man.
Cf. hygiene

Food ionization Treatment of foodstuffs by ionizing radiation with the view to improving their preser-vation.

Food mixture(s) Processed ready to use nutritional food mixture(s) for use in nutritional emergencies.
Cf. corn-soya blend (CSB), corn-soya milk (CSM), instant corn-soya milk (ICSM), K-2 mix, soya-fortified bulghur (SFB), soya-fortified sorghum grits (SFSG), wheat-soya blend (WSB), wheat-soya milk (WSM), yoghourt

Food pattern Data on, or the profile of, the foods consumed by a given community, showing the kinds and amounts of the principal foods eaten at any given time.
Cf. food habits

Food poisoning A general term describing the intestinal and other troubles caused by the ingestion of food or water contaminated by germs, toxic substances and other pathogens, or by an allergic reaction to certain proteins and substances in the food.
Cf. botulism, contamination, toxin

Food ration Cf. ration (food)

Food refrigeration Method of food conservation by maintaining positive temperatures near 0°C, which has the effect of temporarily slowing down microbial and enzymatic processes.
Cf. cold chain

Food relief The provision of foodstuffs on a national or local scale to relieve sudden food shortage and combat malnutrition in a disaster.
Cf. emergency feeding, food aid

Food resources The inventory and stock of foodstuffs available and, in particular, required in an emergency, including the system of storage, warehouse facilities, markets, distribution centres, emergency sources and other food facilities that can be used by the stricken population.

Food safety The component of food hygiene which deals with the measures necessary to ensure the innocuity, cleanliness, salubrity and intrinsic value of foodstuffs.
Cf. food hygiene, foodstuffs, hygiene, food security

Food security Access by all people at all times to enough food for an active, healthy life – World Bank.
Do not confuse with food safety.

Food shortage Situation in which supplies of food available in a country or region are insufficient for the needs. The opposite of food security.

Food taboo A social and/or religious interdiction concerning the handling and consumption of certain foods.

Food-borne disease A general term for disease of infectious bacterial or toxic nature caused by eating a food.
Cf. food-borne intoxication

Food-borne intoxication Disease caused by ingestion of the toxins produced by bacteria.

Food-borne trematode infections A group of parasitic worm infections of liver and lung acquired by eating raw fish, crustaceans and vegetables. Neglected tropical diseases.

Foodstuff Food. Any raw or prepared product which can be consumed by man as food.

Force Meteorology: A numerical expression of the speed of the wind (wind force), or the agitation of the sea (sea force) or of the height of waves.

Cf. Beaufort scale, Douglas scale, wind, wind force, wave

Forecast
1. Description of the meteorological conditions predicted for a given time and over a given zone. Important in disaster prevention.
Sn: weather forecast
2. A statistical estimate or statement concerning a future event (WMO).
Prognosis, prediction and other similar terms are used with varying meanings in various disciplines.

Forel scale Numerical scale indicating the colour of the sea, extending from 0 (deep blue) to 10 (potassium chromate yellow).
Cf. Douglas scale

Forensic geography A field of investigation and detection using legal and technological methods to search and uncover clandestine mass graves (or old historical burial grounds).
Cf. forensic medicine

Forensic medicine The medical specialty that studies and covers all aspects of pathology, disease and death that may possibly, directly or indirectly raise legal issues which need investigation.
Sn: legal medicine

Foreshock(s) Small shakings of the earth's crust preceding the main earthquake in a given area. Also called precursors. The opposite of aftershocks.
Cf. aftershock, earthquake

Forest/vegetation fire(s) Fires in forest, grassland, bush and bushland that usually cover a widespread area and cause extensive damage to property and the environment. They may be due to natural causes, such as lightning or volcanic eruption, may be started illegally by arsonists or carelessly by campers and smokers or may accidentally spread from an intentionally started fire for clearing a forest area.

Disastrous forest fires are quite seasonal in hot, dry regions such as the Mediterranean basin during summer. Widespread and serious air pollution has been caused by huge forest fires in Southeast Asia, with intense accumulation of fine particles that provoke grave respiratory problems.

Sn: vegetation fire(s)

Cf. burn disaster, Mediterranean Council for Burns and Fire Disasters

Forestation Establishment of a forest or plantation of trees, natural or man-made, in an area where a forest was not previously present.

Cf. deforestation, desertification, reforestation, afforestation

Fortified food Food in which the nutritive elements have been intentionally increased or added with the view to improving its nutritional value or to prevent deficiency diseases. Examples: thiamine added to white flour, vitamin D to milk, iodine to salt.

Sn: enriched food

Cf. deficiency disease, food additive, food enrichment, food fortification

Foundation for Innovative New Diagnostics/FIND A Swiss non-profit but also internationally funded organization that works to develop and implement affordable, robust and accurate diagnostic products and technologies.

Fracture Medicine: A break or discontinuity of a bone in the body.

Geology: Fracture zone: Abrupt and massive submarine dislocation of the earth over a long narrow band, where the continuity of the solid structures is interrupted by a transform fault.

Cf. transform fault, sliding fault, earthquake

Fragile State(s) Countries where there is a lack of political commitment, weak governance and/or suffering from violent conflicts that are not conducive to develop and implement needed pro-poor policies. About 50 countries can be thus defined as fragile, its population bearing a disproportionately heavier burden of disease and mortality.

Cf. least developed countries

Fragmentation bomb Bomb that explodes just above ground level, spreading a multiple number of smaller explosives that cause multiple explosions with extensive injuries. Prohibited by international law (Oslo Treaty) and humanitarian standards. Unexploded "bomblets" can persist for a long time, causing a continuing threat.

Sn: cluster bomb

Cf. cluster bomb, law of war, Oslo Treaty

Fratricide effect In nuclear war, the inhibiting effect by X-rays, blast, thermal waves that a nuclear detonation has on the power of a second nuclear weapon on the same target.

Cf. nuclear war

Free pratique In International Health Regulations terminology, it means permission for a ship to enter port, embark or disembark, discharge or load cargo or stores; permission for an aircraft, after landing, to embark or disembark, discharge or load cargo or stores and permission for a ground transport vehicle, upon arrival, to embark or disembark, discharge or load cargo or stores – IHR.

Freedom of opinion Cf. freedom of the press

Freedom of the press Article 19 of the Universal Declaration of Human Rights states: "Everyone has the right to freedom of opinion and expression,… to receive and impart information and ideas through any media and regardless of frontiers". The Declaration of Windhoek, 1991, calls for free, independent and pluralistic media worldwide characterizing free press as essential to democracy and a fundamental human right.
Sn: freedom of speech, freedom of opinion, freedom of expression
Cf. Universal Declaration of Human Rights, Windhoek Declaration

Freedom of speech Cf. freedom of the press, Universal Declaration of Human Rights

Freighting Cf. chartering

French doctors A popular term in English for Médecins sans Frontières, MSF, (Doctors without Borders), a predominantly French voluntary organization of physicians and nurses active in disasters and emergencies throughout the world. Received the Nobel Peace Prize, 1999.
Cf. Médecins sans Frontières, humanitarian medicine, international assistance

Frontal thunderstorm Thunderstorm which occurs at the passage of a climatic front of two air masses.

Frost A fall in the temperature of the air to 0 °C or below, causing freezing on the ground or in the air.

Fujita-Pearson tornado scale A 3-digit scale devised by Fujita (F-scale) and
Pearson (PP scale) that indicates a tornado's intensity (0–5), path length (0–5) and path width (0–7). Abbreviated as FPP scale.
Cf. tornado, Beaufort scale

Fukushima earthquake and nuclear accident On 11 March 2011, at 14:46 h the most powerful earthquake in Japan's history, of over Richter 9 magnitude, shook the Fukushima-Daiichi nuclear power plant area, 250 km northeast of Tokyo, with its epicentre off the east coast of Japan, creating widespread destruction and damaging the complex of six reactors. This was very soon followed by a gigantic tsunami with waves over 20 m, obviously generated by the same tectonic fracture, that reached the Sendai coast and reactor plant site, devastating the surrounding towns and lowlands over many miles. Reactor buildings were further destroyed, caught fire and fuel rods exposed, with partial meltdown. Damage estimated at INES maximum, level 7. Some 30,000 residents were dead, thousands missing or evacuated.
Cf. compound disaster, Three Mile Island, Chernobyl

Fukushima effect At the very time when there was considerable confidence in the safety of nuclear reactors and the nuclear power industry, the disastrous explosion and breakdown of the reactors at Fukushima, Japan, on 11 March 2011, with extensive damage and persistent radioactivity, shook that confidence and has had the effect of several countries rethinking their nuclear projects and exploring other sources of energy. Many have decreed a moratorium
Switzerland and Germany have decided, by law, to abandon further plans and to dismantle and decommission all their existing plants by about 2030.

Cf. Fukushima nuclear disaster, nuclear dismantling/decommissioning, disaster legislation, technological disaster

Full-cream milk powder Sn: dried full-cream milk, dried whole milk, DFCM, DWM

Full-scope safeguards In the nuclear industry, supervision by the International Atomic Energy Authority of all nuclear facilities in a State with the aim of ensuring that fissionable material is not utilized for weapon's manufacture and that it is also otherwise safe.
Cf. arms control. IAEA

Fumigation The process of dispersion of fine gaseous particles of chemical agents used to kill harmful animal species, such as insects.
Cf. disinfestation

Fund for Armenian Relief/FAR Emergency fund raised in the USA to aid the victims of the 1988 devastating earthquake at Spitak, Armenia, great numbers of whom continue needing neurosurgical, orthopaedic, general social and health assistance and rebuilding still insufficient. Hundred and eleven nations have responded to this exceptional disaster.
Cf. Spitak earthquake

Fund raising Appeal soliciting contributions and seeking money for a humanitarian cause.
Cf. donor agency, request for disaster assistance

Fundamentalism Extremely strict observance of traditional principles and tenets of holy scriptures of a faith, e.g. the Bible, Talmud or Quran, held and interpreted by certain adepts of that faith to be fundamental and beyond any challenge.

Fungicide Medicament or chemical compound used to treat fungal infections and to kill fungus.

Cf. pesticide

Fusion bomb Nuclear weapon in which the explosive power (other than the triggering by fission) is derived from the fusion of the light nuclei, liberating energy and radiation. There are also nuclear weapons which use a three-stage release of energy – fission, fusion, fission (Cf. FFF bomb).
Sn: hydrogen bomb, thermonuclear bomb
Cf. atom bomb, fission bomb, nuclear war

G

G-20 countries Twenty of the richest, industrialized and emerging countries, representing about 90% of the gross national product of the world.
Cf. developing countries

Gabion An anti-erosion device consisting of a wire box filled with stones, retaining the soil in slope while allowing the water to drain away.
Cf. erosion

Gale Violent wind of force 8 or 9 on the Beaufort scale. Between 34 and 40 knots.
Cf. Beaufort scale, cyclone, hurricane, storm, typhoon

Gale warning Meteorological message intended to warn those concerned of the existence or expected occurrence of a wind of Beaufort force 8 or 9 over a specified area.
Cf. Beaufort scale

Gamma rays Electromagnetic radiation of very short wavelength and high energy, composed of photons emitted by the nuclei of certain radionuclides and accompanying many nuclear reactions, such as fission.
Cf. fission, radionuclide

Gates Foundation Cf. Bill and Melinda Gates Foundation

Gender In humans, generally refers to the masculine or feminine sex. In society, however, gender refers to the socially established sex roles, values, attributes, customs and expectations that society ascribes to one or the other sex in the community. There should be no gender discrimination. Cf. gender mainstreaming

Gender mainstreaming The process of assessing the implications for women and men of any planned action, including legislation, policies or programmes, in all areas and at all levels. It is a strategy for making women's as well as men's concerns and experiences an integral dimension of the design, implementation, monitoring and evaluation of policies and programmes in all political, economic and social spheres so that women and men benefit equally, and inequality is not perpetuated. The ultimate aim is to achieve gender equality – ECOSOC.

Generic drug Non-proprietary medicament prescribed and sold under its chemical name rather than a trade brand name. Usually cheaper than a proprietary mark.

Genetic effects/aberration Abnormal changes in the germ cells caused by toxic pollutants or radiation. Sn: chromosomal aberration Cf. Chernobyl, chromosome, radioactive contamination, Seveso, technological disaster, thalidomide

Genetics The field of biological science that deals with the phenomena and mechanisms of heredity. Genetic problems may occur following toxic and radioactive disasters.

Cf. radioactive contamination, technological disaster.

Geneva Conventions (Red Cross) The body of international agreements consisting of four Conventions (1949) and two Additional Protocols (1977), concerning humanitarian treatment of victims of armed conflict and put under the responsibility of the International Committee of the Red Cross. The first Protocol regulates the care of the wounded and sick soldiers on the battlefield; the second is about the care of the wounded, sick and shipwrecked in naval warfare; the third on the treatment of prisoners of war and the fourth on the protection of civilians in time of war. Additional Protocols I and II ensure more humane consideration not only in international conflicts but also in national strife, such as the treatment of guerrilla fighters. (Note: Possible additional protocols are being considered to meet the changing needs in the twenty-first century.)
Cf. International Humanitarian Law, Red Cross, human rights, humanitarian medicine

Geneva Protocol (chemical and bacteriological weapons) Protocol for the Prohibition of the Use in War of Asphyxiating, Poisonous or other Gases and of Bacteriological Methods of Warfare (1925). It prohibits the use in war of asphyxiating poisonous or other gases and of bacteriological weapons. While prohibiting the use, it does not, however, forbid the development, production, stockpiling or deployment of chemical or biological weapons. Another weakness is that it provides no procedures against violations.

The 1975 Biological Weapons Convention complements the 1925 Geneva Protocol in that besides the previous prohibitions, it goes a step further in mandating the destruction of such weapons and their conversion to peaceful purposes.
Cf. biological warfare, chemical weapons, biological weapons, BCW

Geneva summit (Cold War) The meeting in Geneva, Switzerland, in 1985, between Ronald Reagan, President of the United States, and Mikhail Gorbachev, General Secretary of the Central Committee of the Communist Party of the USSR, a historic encounter between two enemies and opposing political systems that marked the beginning of the end of the post-World War II Cold War.

Genital mutilation Cf. female genital mutilation, excision, infibulation, introcision

Geneva University/Geneva city By history, tradition and by proximity to the UN, Red Cross and other international institutions, the city, the University and the Geneva Hospitals (HUG) have long been involved in international work, with a Division of International and Humanitarian Health, a Foundation for Education (GFMER), an annual Health Forum (GHF), GIPRI, Graduate Institute, etc.

Genocide Any of the following acts committed with intent to destroy, in whole or in part, national, ethnic, racial or religious groups, e.g. (a) killing members of the group, (b) causing serious bodily or mental harm to the group, (c) deliberately inflicting conditions of life calculated to cause the group's total or partial destruction, (d) imposing measures to prevent births and (f) forcibly transferring children

to another group. The following shall be punishable: genocide; conspiracy, attempt and incitement to commit genocide, complicity in genocide – ICC. Examples: Armenians by Turks in 1915, Nazi extermination of Jews 1938–1944, Tutsis by Hutus in Rwanda 1994 – J. Last.
Cf. crimes against humanity, deportation, ethnic cleansing, human rights, International Criminal Court, man-conceived disaster, torture, Universal Declaration of Human Rights

Geodetic A geographic and mathematical science that seeks to define the shape of the earth and that determines the areas and different points on the earth's topographic surface in relation to a reference system.
Cf. topography

Geographic information systems Traditional maps and more elaborate computer programmes that reflect relevant data and analyses on a part of the earth that is being investigated for communication and disaster management purposes.
Sn: GIS

Geographic longitude Angular distance of any point on the earth's surface, longitudinal lines east or west of a standard meridian (0 °) situated at Greenwich.
Sn: longitude, terrestrial longitude
Cf. latitude

Geological hazard(s) Earth movements or unstable natural land phenomena that may constitute a risk or cause damage to property, the built environment, the socioeconomic fabric or injury and death.

Geomorphology The science concerned with the earth's surface and the evolution of the globe's relief features.

Ghetto/Ghettoization Originally a restricted area in fifteenth-century Venice, it now denotes an unpopular, circumscribed slum or poor section in a city. Ghettoization is the forceful confining of a minority group into a designated area.
Cf. slum, favela, discrimination

Glasgow coma scale/GCS Coma is unconsciousness. The scale is a practical means of assessing changes in the level of responsiveness in the unconscious, comatose or severely injured person. Three systems are monitored; in the eye, the result may be (a) no response, (b) response to pain, (c) to verbal command, (d) opens eye spontaneously. The total score for a positive degree of consciousness is between 3 and 15.
Cf. trauma score

Glasnost Russian word for transparency. An attempt to reform and democratize the secretive Soviet regime towards the end of its reign.
Cf. transparency, Transparency International

Glasshouse effect In addition to natural heat release from the earth into the atmosphere, there is increasing industrial, man-made heat production (combustion of coal, petroleum and natural gas) releasing the gas carbon dioxide (CO_2) into the atmosphere. While CO_2 is essentially transparent to incoming solar energy, it is not transparent to re-radiated energy emitted by the earth itself. Thus, a heating process referred to as the "glasshouse" or "hothouse" effect is produced, with wide-scale environmental consequences. Sn: hothouse phenomenon, greenhouse effect
Cf. atmospheric pollution, ozone depletion, chlorofluorocarbons, global warming, Kyoto protocol, climate change, CO_2

GLAWARS Commission Report The extensive investigation carried out by the Greater London Area War Risk Study Commission on the likely effects of modern warfare on a major metropolitan centre like London. Published under the title "London Under Attack", its conclusions have been found applicable to most modern urban centres, translated into Italian under the title of "Attacco alla Città".
Cf. WHOPAX Report, armed conflict, civil defence, nuclear war

Global Academy of Tropical Health and Cultural Development/GATH Organization promoting and involved in total health care in tropical areas with a particular view of cultural factors.

Global Alliance for Improved Nutrition/GAIN Child malnutrition is a global problem, especially in developing countries. This non-profit organization fights against malnutrition, for food fortification and improved infant and child nutrition for better health.

Global Alliance for Vaccines and Immunization/GAVI An international, interagency enterprise to promote vaccine development and delivery, particularly in low-income countries. A coalition of the Bill and Melinda Gates Foundation, World Bank, WHO, UNICEF and NGOs.
Cf. global compact

Global compact United Nations partnership with business and the private sector as legitimate and fruitful partners particularly in the public health field, e.g. with Roche Pharmaceuticals or the Bill and Melinda Gates Foundation.
Cf. global alliance

Global Earth Observation System of Systems/GEOSS A mainly inter-governmental technical partnership of GEO (Group on Earth Observations) for an international system to reduce damage from disasters, to better understand the weather and environmental effects on health, to support agriculture and combat desertification.

Global fallout Cf. fallout

Global Forum for Health Research/ GFHR Affiliated but not a part of WHO, the independent Global Forum strives to narrow the financing gap that disadvantages research for diseases of poor countries. The 10/90 gap.

Global frequency Term used for prevalence, but not recommended.
Cf. prevalence

Global Fund to Fight AIDS, Tuberculosis and Malaria An extensive, long-term multimillion dollar fund initiated primarily by WHO, UNAIDS and the Gates Foundation to provide long-term medication and sustained treatment for AIDS, tuberculosis and malaria. It is an innovative, cooperative funding approach aiming at increasing the finances and resources against global, devastating diseases, initially beginning with the three mentioned above.
Sn: referred to as the Global Fund
Cf. global health partnership

Global health More than international health, global health refers to health issues both at the geographic global level and the disease global level, in that it considers health and disease not limited to borders or nations, and disease not limited to bacteriology or other pathologic considerations only. It transcends these and takes into account also such non-medical economic and political interactions and interdependence as poverty and mortality, GDP and disease, level of education and health.
Cf. international health, Health for All, Millennium Development Goals, World Health Organization

Global Health Cluster/WHO An aggregate of international, national and organizational experts working at the global, regional and country levels to strengthen the humanitarian action of WHO.

Global health diplomacy Policy-shaping processes through which States, intergovernmental organizations and non-State actors negotiate responses to health challenges or utilize health concepts or mechanisms in policy shaping and negotiation strategies to achieve other political, economic or social objectives – Carleton University GHD.

Global health partnership Various forms of cooperative work with the view to scientifically, financially and organizationally tackling a specific or a variety of health problems. Example: GAVI

Good Humanitarian Donorship/ GHD In 2003, donor governments proclaimed a Declaration of Good Humanitarian Donorship outlining a series of criteria concerning the timeliness, quality and effectiveness of their humanitarian assistance policies, funding and practices.
Cf. humanitarian response index, development assistance research associates, aid

Global Observing System An extensive system of techniques and facilities of World Weather Watch for recording weather observations on a worldwide scale.

Syn: GOS
Cf. WWW, World Meteorological Organization

Global Public Health Intelligence Network A collaborative network between Canada and WHO involving an Internet-based international early warning system for communicable disease outbreaks (GPHIN).
Cf. pandemic

Global public good A public service with benefits that is strongly universal in terms of countries (more than one group of countries), people (benefiting several, preferably all population groups) and generations (both current and future, without limiting options for future generations) – GFHR/WHO.

Global warming General warming of the earth's surface temperature by small but significant degrees, due, besides natural phenomena, to such man-made factors as industrial gas emissions, petroleum production, ozone depletion, atmospheric pollution, resulting in harmful effects that disturb the global climatic equilibrium and can lead to disaster. A global warming of between 1.5 and 4.5 °C is expected to result in sea level rises of up to 20–40 cm, leading to an increase in severity and frequency of floods, submerging of coastal areas and inundation of productive lands.
Cf. chlorofluorocarbons, El Niňo, glasshouse effects, Kyoto protocol, ozone depletion, World Meteorological Organization, CO_2

Globalization The expansion worldwide, through a liberal market economy model, of the infrastructures of commerce, communication, information and other sectors of societal organization, making the globe "smaller" but with varying (positive and negative) effects on the social, health and developmental activities of people throughout the world.

Glowing avalanche A form of ash flow, resulting from incandescent tephra streaming along the slopes of the volcano.
Cf. ash flow, tephra, volcano

Glowing cloud Burning mixture of volcanic gas and suspended solid particles falling by gravity and by pressure of gases along the flanks of the erupting volcano.
Sn: "Nuée ardente"
Cf. ash flow, volcano, falling cloud

Goal A defined aim towards which to strive and the actions taken to achieve it. Example: The goal may be to have an environment that is conducive to health or to have primary health care available to everybody in a refugee settlement. A global effort is the United Nations programme of Millennium Development Goals 2000–2015 (Cf.)
Cf. objective, plan, target, MDGs

GOES satellite Cf. SMS/GOES satellites

Goitre, goiter Benign and diffuse enlargement of the thyroid gland due to lack of iodine, endemic in certain areas of the world.
Cf. basal metabolic rate, endemic disease, deficiency disease, iodine, Lugol's iodine, thyroid

Gonorrhoea Sexually transmitted disease due to *Neisseria gonorrhoeae*, usually manifested by urethritis in men, vaginitis or cervicitis in women and ophthalmia in infants.
Cf. sexually transmitted disease

Good manufacturing practice WHO guidelines and model "designed to ensure that products are consistently produced and controlled according to a specific set of quality standards to

avoid contamination, incorrect label-
ling and inappropriate levels of active
ingredients" – GMP/WHO.

Governance Term usually interchange-
able with government, but recently
increasingly used to denote the mechanisms, manner, system, strong points,
weak points and functioning of governing in action.
Cf. government

Government Body or office of persons,
elected or non-elected, and the rules,
authority and responsibility attached
thereto that makes decisions for,
governs or administers a State.
Cf.   governance,   democracy,
dictatorship

Graduate Institute, Geneva More correctly, the Graduate Institute of
International Development Studies
(Institut de Hautes Etudes Internationales et du Développement,
IHEID), a higher academic institution
that carries out studies and provides
courses on international law, political
science and development, as well as on
global health and health diplomacy.

Gray A much used but ill-clarified term,
not defined in the Geneva Conventions.
It refers to a war between organized
armed insurgent opposition groups
and the regular armed forces within
the same nation or State. A recent
definition is 'non-international armed
conflict'.
Cf. war, armed conflict, guerilla,
Geneva Conventions

**Great Hanshin-Awaji earth-
quake** Extensively devastating
earthquake that struck the Kobe
(Japan) area on 17 January 1995,
killing over 6,400 people and injur-
ing about 40,000. Cf. also the
Fukushima earthquake.

Green Cross International/GCI
Humanitarian organization initiated
by Mikhail Gorbachev, Nobel Peace
Laureate, to promote conflict resolution, healthy environment, peace and
upholding human values in society.

Greenhouse gas A gas, such as carbon
dioxide (CO_2), methane, chlorofluorocarbons (CFCs) and hydro-
chlorofluorocarbons, (HCFCs) that
absorbs and re-emits infrared radiation, warming the earth's surface
and contributing to climate change.
– UNEP. Abbreviated as GHG.
Cf. greenhouse gas, hothouse phenomenon, climate change

Greenpeace Independent worldwide
organization that upholds respect for
– and exposes breaches of – action by
industries, governments or people that
pollute and degrade the environment,
e.g. the deterioration of the oceans,
destruction of ancient forests, global
warming, nuclear threat. Also active
in promoting peace and human rights.
Cf. environmental pollution, climate
change, nuclear war

Greenwich Mean Time Universal coordinated standard reference time based
on the time at the Royal Observatory
in Greenwich, England, at 0° longitude. Usually referred to as GMT. To
the West of Greenwich, the hour is
–GMT, and to the East, +GMT.
Sn: GMT, universal coordinated time,
Zulu time

Gross domestic product The total value
of all goods and services produced
within a given country, irrespective of
ownership. Abbreviated as GDP. The
term is being increasingly replaced by
Gross National Product, GNP.
Cf. Gross national product

Gross national product The total value of
all goods and services produced in a

country during a given period, usually a year, expressed in monetary terms, at current prices, produced and owned by the nation's citizens. Abbreviated as GNP.

Cf. Gross domestic product

Ground level concentration Sn: concentration (of a toxic or radioactive material) at ground level.

Ground swell Popular expression describing solitary high wave(s).

Groundwater level The level at which underground water saturates the overlying rock and soil.

Ground zero Sn: hypocentre (nuclear explosion)

Cf. zone zero

Groupe de Bellerive An independent forum for rational and unbiased discussion by socially conscious, highly respectable scientists, statesmen and thinkers, on major issues facing humanity, such as peace, security, nuclear risk, disarmament, environment, international terrorism, renewable energy or human interdependence.

Guardian A person who has or has been entrusted with the legal authority and decisional power over a child, minor, seriously sick patient or incompetent person, for the advantage of that person.

Cf. unaccompanied minor

Guerrilla Literally "small war", which takes on a different meaning or interpretation according to whether it is justified or unjustified, struggle for independence, liberation, resistance or insurrection, destruction and subjugation. In International humanitarian law, the Geneva Conventions and United Nations instruments have difficulty in dealing with such situations.

Cf. International humanitarian law, Geneva Conventions, conflict, armed conflict, kamikaze, civil war

Gulbenkian Foundation Primarily founded to rescue and alleviate the sufferings of the Armenian people from the massacres of 1915–1917, this benevolent organization has now expanded into education and the prestigious fields of art (G. Museum), music (G. Orchestra) and human welfare, based in Portugal.

Gulf War syndrome Condition observed in soldiers who served in the Gulf War, 1961, characterized by general fatigue, pain in the limbs and general depression. Exposure to chemical weapons and depleted uranium has been suspected.

Gust Sn: squall

Gypsies Cf. tziganes, Roma, nomad, population mobility, racism

H

Habitat

1. The ecological frame and dwelling place to which a species or community is adapted.
2. The space occupied by man for his domestic life and related activities.
3. Shortened name for the United Nations Centre for Human Settlements.

Habituation The process by which an organism (or society) becomes gradually accustomed and insensitive to certain changes in the environment.

The term is also used for addiction, substance dependence and excessive drug consumption.

Cf. environment, society

Hacking The secret, unauthorized, illegal penetration by unobtrusive cyberelectronic means into a computer data base, telephone or other network with the view to disrupting, damaging, destroying or acquiring information.

Halal Arabic word for lawful. Food that is permissible to eat according to Islamic law. Opposite of Haram.
Cf. sharia, custom, kosher

Half-life Cf. radioactive half-life

Ham radio An amateur radio used for two-way communications usually as a private hobby, but the international network of which can be quite useful in disaster situations.
Cf. International Telecommunication Union

Handicap A congenital or acquired diminution of varying degrees, in a person's ability to perform a mental, physical, occupational or social function.

Harassing agents Chemical substances that are used to temporarily harass crowds or control riots, as with tear gases. Risky as they are, these chemicals are not considered as lethal weapons in conventional war and their use is not prohibited. For example, they are often used by the police.
Cf. tear gas, lethal agent, incapacitating agent, chemical weapons, war

Harnessing Cf. water harnessing

Hawaiian type eruption Nonexplosive volcanic action producing a creeping lava flow with low gas pressure, solidifying in layers as it creeps and sometimes forming an incandescent lake.
Cf. volcano, creep

Hazard The probability of the occurrence of a disaster caused by a natural phenomenon (earthquake, cyclone) or by failure of man-made sources of energy (nuclear reactor, industrial explosion) or by uncontrolled human activity (overgrazing, heavy traffic, conflicts) – UN.
Potential source of harm – ISO.
Some authors use the term in a broader sense, including vulnerability, elements at risk and the consequences of risk.

Cf. elements at risk, natural hazard, risk, vulnerability, secondary hazard

Hazard analysis Investigation, study and monitoring of a hazard with the view to identifying its origin, behaviour, characteristics and damage potential.

Hazard classification Cf. UN hazard classification

Hazard mapping Cf. zoning

Hazardous area An area, building or facility with more than usual fire risks, structural collapse, flooding, chemical contamination, etc. It may also refer to a particular part of a building, such as the radiation laboratory in a hospital.

Hazardous material A substance, gaseous, liquid or solid, such as a toxic chemical, that has been designated by the appropriate authorities as being potentially dangerous to health, safety or property, and the handling and transport of which are subjected to strict legislation.
Sn: hazmat
Cf. UN hazard classification, Basel Convention, hazard analysis

Hazmat Abbreviation for hazardous material.

H-bomb Sn: hydrogen bomb

Health
1. The state of complete physical, mental and social well-being and not merely the absence of disease or infirmity – WHO.
2. The state of an individual or a community free from disabilitating conditions and harassing circumstances, demonstrating a reasonable resistance to diseases and living in a salubrious environment.

Health-care levels Cf. Primary health care, secondary health care, tertiary health care

Health centre A facility from which health care is delivered to a defined community or area. It is a centre that carries out promotive, protective, preventive, diagnostic, curative and rehabilitative activities for ambulant people. Normally, it has no beds – WHO. In some countries, the scope of such a centre may be wider.

Health development The process of continuous, progressive improvement of health status of a population – WHO. And all the activities undertaken in respect of such improvement.

Health diplomacy Cf. global health diplomacy, diplomacy, humanitarian diplomacy

Health education The approaches and techniques used to promote sanitary living habits in the community and to inculcate knowledge and practices of hygienic behaviour in individuals as the basic element of primary health care within personal and national development. Not to be confused with medical education.

Health in all policies principle In strengthening the philosophy of Health for All, a new emphasis based on the principle that peoples' health can be improved through policies that are mainly controlled by sectors other than health.
Cf. Millennium Development Goals, health diplomacy

Health promotion The aggregate of educational, advocacy, informative and demonstration processes to encourage and enable people to increase their control over and ameliorate their health.
Cf. health diplomacy

Health research Systematic qualitative and quantitative investigation to enhance the understanding of health and its application both in the field of disease-causing pathogens as well as in the wider determinants of global health, including environmental, social, economic and political elements.

Health resources Inventory of medical and related personnel, of health workers, services, hospitals and clinics, public and private medical and drug supplies, pharmaceutical distributors with records of stocks of medicines and vaccines and other health facilities.
Cf. health workers

Health sustainability Providing a system of health that responds to current needs, maintains that level and does not encroach upon the health needs of future generations.
Cf. sustainability

Health system A system that consists of organizations, people and actions whose primary intent is to promote, restore and maintain health, with the goals of improving health and health equity in ways that are responsive, financially fair and make the best or most efficient use of available resources – WHO.

Health transition In a given population, variations in the underlying causes of disease and death that stem from changes in the interrelated elements of demographic structure, epidemiological patterns, geographic changes and transition risk factors.

Health workers All persons engaged in actions whose primary intent is to enhance health – WHO.

Heat illness Exposure to high temperatures can cause heat-related illness in the form of heat cramps, heat exhaustion, heat stroke, exertional heat sickness, skin injury due to extreme sunburn, etc. Heat illness occurs when the body generates, or is exposed to, more heat than it can dissipate.

In tropical countries and open refugee communities, the people suffer less as their body is adjusted to such temperatures, while expatriate relief workers can be quite ill from heat and humidity. Heat stroke. (Not to confuse with burn disease.)

Heavy water Deuterium oxide, or water containing a high proportion of deuterium atoms, HDO or D_2O

Heimlich manoeuvre An emergency, on site non-invasive manoeuvre to liberate an obstructed airway by applying immediate, sudden and firm pressure on the upper abdomen that helps eject the blocking object.

Helminthiasis A variety of diseases caused by the presence of parasitic worms (helminths) in the body. Usually soil-transmitted. Common in poor and crowded conditions.
Cf. parasitic diseases

Helsinki Conference 2005 International conference held in 2005 in Helsinki, Finland, with the aim of engaging parliamentarians to foster accountability in global institutions, to meet the promises of the UN Millennium Development Goals and to formulate effective measures to tackle global health crises.
Cf. accountability, Millennium Development Goals

Helsinki Declaration A formal statement made in 1964 by WHO and the World Medical Association (WMA) that establishes 12 ethical principles to all scientists and health personnel on research and experimentation involving human subjects. In particular, it imposes the necessity of informed consent by the patient and extends the Nuremberg Code.
Cf. Nuremberg Code, informed consent, ethics

Hepatitis Any inflammation of the liver due to infection, allergy or toxic substances. Includes acute viral hepatitis (A, B) and other types (C).
Cf. viral hepatitis (A, B, C).

Herbicide Chemical compound used to kill undesirable plants and weeds. In chemical warfare, it is used as a weapon to kill vegetation.
Cf. chemical warfare, defoliant, pesticide, agent orange

Hero Acronymic term for hazard of electromagnetic radiation to ordnance.
CF. electromagnetic pulse/EMP

Heroism Courageous conduct beyond the call of duty, often putting one's life in danger in the process of helping another. Noble act, not infrequently seen at the site of a disaster and in humanitarian work.

High Commissioner for Human Rights Cf. Office of the High Commissioner for Human Rights, United Nations

High-income countries The World Bank categorizes (2008) according to gross national income (GNI, previously GNP) per capita: high-income countries: US$11,906 or more.
Sn: developed countries, industrialized countries
Cf. upper-middle income countries, low-income countries, country income classification

High-pressure area Sn: anticyclone

High-pressure ridge Extension of a high-pressure zone in a less elevated zone.
Cf. atmospheric pressure, anticyclone

High seas
1. That part of the sea that is out of vision from the coast.
2. Waters situated beyond the territorial sea and free of any sovereignty.

The "Boat people" were attacked on the high seas outside Vietnam.

Sn: open sea Cf. piracy

Hijacking An illegal violent action committed mainly in an airplane, sometimes on the highway, for private, criminal or political ends.

Cf. piracy

Hiroshima/Nagasaki Industrial cities in Japan. Hiroshima was the first ever human settlement to be attacked with an atomic bomb, at 8:15 a.m., on 6 August 1945, towards the end of World War II, resulting in massive destruction, radioactive fallout, immediate massacre with 80,000 civilian deaths, more than 210,000 victims and long-lasting health and radioactivity consequences that are still continuing. The bomb was of uranium type, equivalent to 13,000 tons of TNT.

Nagasaki was targeted on 9 August, with a plutonium type bomb. The only two cities to date to have been subjected to atomic attacks.

Cf. atom bomb, nuclear war, uranium, plutonium, crimes against humanity

Holistic medicine A health and disease perception of good medicine based on the principle that the whole (wholistic) person in his environment should be treated rather than merely the disease or injured part.

Holistic recovery (disaster) A holistic recovery from disaster is one in which the stricken locality systematically considers each of the principles of sustainability in every decision it makes about reconstruction and redevelopment – Nat. Hazard.

Holocaust Literally means burning to complete destruction. Historically a horrible and totally condemnable policy of certain governments against target populations, with intent to annihilate them, e.g. the Spanish colonizers against the Maya and Aztec, Nazis against Jews.

Cf. genocide, human rights, man-conceived disaster

Homosexuality The biological sex instinct normally induces attraction and attachment between man and woman (heterosexual). A small minority feel differently, to a person of the same sex (homosexual) or to either sex (bisexual). The usual term for men is "gay" and for women is "lesbian". These should not be discriminated against.

Hookworm Sn: ankylostomiasis

Horizontal transmission Disease transmission from one person to another in the same generation, as opposed to transmission from one generation to another, e.g. HIV transmission from mother to baby.

Hospice A well-intentioned institution or other facility that provides palliative care for the incurably sick, terminally ill or the dying.

Hospital capacity (in mass casualty situation) In a mass casualty situation, with many patients arriving at the same time, the theoretical capacity of a hospital would be its ability to admit or manage a number of victims amounting to approximately 20% of its normal bed capacity.

Cf. mass casualty situation, casualty

Hospitalization in disasters Cf. mass casualty situation

Host country Country or its government where a refugee, asylum seeker or disaster victim is accepted and receives humanitarian assistance.

Hostage Person abducted by force and held against his will, usually for political pressure or monetary gain.

Hothouse phenomenon Sn: glasshouse effects, greenhouse effect
Cf. global warming, ozone depletion, climate change

Hotline A telephone number or other direct communication method accessible during emergencies or for other useful information, such as police, fire, civil defence.
Cf. civil defence, alarm

Household A family or several persons forming a domestic commonalty, living under the same roof.
Sn: household unit
Cf. community

Household survey Any study or enquiry which is based on household samples. For example, food consumer surveys, preference surveys, demographic surveys.
Cf. food consumption survey, socio-economic survey

Housing The act of providing a person with shelter or temporary lodgings.
Sn: sheltering

Human development Progress of individuals – and by extension of their community – towards fulfilment of their manual, intellectual and cultural capacities and of their personal potentialities.
Cf. development, sustainable development

Human failure (accident/error/disaster) A disaster caused or aggravated by a human deficiency or due to a human factor. "It is estimated that as a direct loss-causing agent human failure accounts for about 15% of all accidents", the rate varying according to several parameters. The main parameters controlling human failure are the aggregate of (a) the ability, qualification and awareness of the participating expert(s); (b) the residual chance of human failure; (c) knowledge of the problem; (d) training received by the person(s) concerned; (e) experience of the person(s) concerned; (f) risk awareness of the person(s) concerned; (g) motivation of these persons to prevent accident and (h) the personal risk to the individual should an accident occur. The effects of these parameters often overlap – Tiedemann, Swiss Re.

Human immunodeficiency virus (HIV) The causal organism of AIDS.
Sn: HIV Cf. AIDS, immunodeficiency

Human rights The inalienable rights of every human being, based on the recognition by all of the inherent dignity and equality of each person, as codified and guaranteed by the Universal Declaration of Human Rights, Convention européenne des Droits de l'Homme, and other international instruments.
Sn: sometimes called the Rights of Man (especially in French).
Cf. High Commissioner for Human Rights, humanitarian medicine, International Association for Humanitarian Medicine, International Criminal Court, Universal Declaration of Human Rights, humanitarian, absolute human right, UNHCHR

Human Rights, Universal Declaration of Cf. Universal Declaration of Human Rights

Human security A desirable and essential condition in which man's freedom from fear and from want are ensured. Safety from disease, hunger and violence are corollaries.

Human settlement An organized system of varying size – from village to metropolis – which englobes in one functional whole the community, its habitat and its activities.

Cf. habitat, community, HABITAT/ UN

Human shield The use of a person as a safety shield, whether that person is a man, woman or child, civilian or soldier, injured or healthy, prisoner-of-war or health worker.

Holding a human shield constitutes a crime of war.

Humane Possessing the higher human qualities of compassion, love, benevolence, caring and sharing, as befits a finer person.

Humanitarian Concept: The view that a person's and humane society's beliefs and actions should benefit mankind, its advancement and its benevolent values.

Action: Work and services undertaken for the advancement and the welfare of humanity without regard to race, religion, politics or profit.

Adjective: Relating to or of a beneficial action or humanitarian aims. Compassionate.

Under some conflict circumstances, allowable humanitarian aid may be limited to basic needs of food, health and shelter.

Cf. International Humanitarian Law, Universal Declaration of Human Rights, UNHCHR, OHCHR, IAHM

Humanitarian action Any work, service, advocacy or assistance of moral, legal, professional, social or physical nature, provided to a person or community, within the concepts of the Universal Declaration of Human Rights and the United Nations actions, to safeguard and uphold the fundamental rights of a person and human society. Also any action

needed to fight against the breach of human rights.

Cf. humanitarian, Universal Declaration of Human Rights, International Association for Humanitarian Medicine, UNHCHR, humanitarian health action, OCHA

Humanitarian assistance/relief Aid or relief of any kind, extent or amount, offered voluntarily to persons or communities suffering from any cause, in the spirit of compassion, humanity, impartiality, neutrality and without any consideration of gain. Funding gives precedence to people-focused survival and basic needs programmes, with special consideration to the human rights dimension of health, especially in vulnerable groups.

Cf. aid, humanitarian, humanitarian medicine, international assistance, International Association for Humanitarian Medicine, Red Cross, relief

Humanitarian assistance by governments. Efficacy score in 2011 Out of 23 donor countries, the following ten proved the most effective in their humanitarian aid in 2011, as based on the DARA criteria: (1) Norway, (2) Denmark, (3) Sweden, (4) Ireland, (5) the Netherlands, (6) Switzerland, (7) European Commission, (8) United Kingdom, (9) Finland, (10) Australia – *Le Temps.*

Cf. development assistance research associates, humanitarian response index, good humanitarian donorship

Humanitarian Charter and Standards Humanitarian Charter and Minimum Standards in Disaster Response. A declaration of principles by several non-governmental organizations (the Sphere Group) aiming at increasing the effectiveness of humanitarian assistance and making humanitarian agencies more accountable in disaster response. The Charter affirms the fundamental importance of (a) the right to life with dignity, (b) distinction between combatants and non-combatants and (c) the principle of non-refoulement. The Standards also set minimal (but not exclusive) requirements for (a) water supply and sanitation, (b) nutrition, (c) food aid, (d) shelter and (e) health services.

Cf. humanitarian, humanitarian medicine, humanitarian assistance

Humanitarian corridor A temporary combat-free passage agreed to by belligerents for safe humanitarian access to evacuate the wounded and besieged and provide food.

Humanitarian diplomacy The process of persuading decision-makers and opinion leaders to act, at all times, in the interests of vulnerable people and with full respect for fundamental humanitarian principles – IFRC Red Cross.

Cf. global health diplomacy, humanitarian medicine, IAHM

Humanitarian health action A single or aggregate of actions performed towards the fulfilment of the principle of the right to health and actions in situations where health is in jeopardy.

Cf. humanitarian assistance

Humanitarian intervention Cf. right to intervene, le droit d'ingérence

Humanitarian Law Correct appellation: International Humanitarian Law (Cf.). Refers principally to the Red Cross Conventions law of armed conflict or law of war, not to be confused with other humanitarian legislation, the UNHCHR or OHCHR.

Sn: law of war

Cf. law of war, International Humanitarian Law, Red Cross Conventions

Humanitarian medicine While all medical intervention to reduce a person's sickness and suffering is in essence humanitarian, humanitarian medicine goes beyond the usual therapeutic act and promotes, provides, teaches, supports and delivers people's health as a human right, in conformity with the ethics of Hippocratic teaching, the principles of the World Health Organization, the Charter of the United Nations, the Universal Declaration of Human Rights, the Red Cross Conventions and other covenants and practices that ensure the most humane and best possible level of care, without any discrimination or consideration of material gain – Gunn.

Cf. humanitarian, International Association for Humanitarian Medicine, International Humanitarian Law, Geneva Conventions, Universal Declaration of Human Rights, World Health Organization

Humanitarian principle The principle that all men are equal and that all human beings shall enjoy the basic necessities of life, adequate health and security, prevention and alleviation of suffering, protection of well-being, their human rights and respect for dignity.

Cf. basic needs, human rights, Universal Declaration of Human Rights

Humanitarian response criteria Cf. humanitarian response index, good humanitarian donorship, DARA, humanitarian assistance by governments, Sphere Project

Humanitarian Response Index (HRI) Humanitarian assistance may be assessed in different ways. One method is that of the Sphere Project (Cf.). DARA International has set a Humanitarian Response Index based on five criteria: (1) responding to needs; (2) prevention, risk reduction and recovery; (3) working with humanitarian partners; (4) protection and international law; (5) learning and accountability.

Cf. Development assistance research associates, Sphere Project, aid, humanitarian charter, good humanitarian donorship, humanitarian assistance by governments

Humanitarian surgery The provision of any or all of the following surgical services by a person or group: the occasional surgical actions needed unexpectedly and provided *pro bono* and without personal advantage or a long-term action dedicated to charitable surgical efforts rather than routine surgical practice, a career devoted to missionary surgery, the provision of surgical care to the underserved or of essential surgery to developing countries under difficult conditions, or of educational programmes with the view to strengthening the surgical capacity in such countries.

Cf. humanitarian medicine, essential surgery, Surgeons OverSeas, International Association for Humanitarian Medicine, American College of Surgeons, Royal College of Surgeons of Canada

Humanitarian war An unacceptable, illogical term, sometimes used for humanitarian intervention or the right to intervene. Term not to be used.

Hunger The physical and mental complex of unpleasant sensations provoked by deprivation of food and relieved by the ingestion of food. Food shortages result in mass hunger.

Cf. famine, food, the Hunger Project

Hunger strike An extreme expression of protest by self-imposed starvation, prolonged refusal of any food, usually to obtain release, acceptance of one's cause or promote a political ideology.

Hurricane A tropical cyclone of wind force 12 on the Beaufort scale, i.e. more than 58 knots. Hurricanes of the West Indies, Western Pacific typhoons and Bay of Bengal cyclones are essentially the same phenomenon; now, all tend to be called tropical cyclones. (Sn.)

Cf. Beaufort scale, Saffir-Simpson scale, cyclone, gale, typhoon, tropical cyclone

Hurricane warning Meteorological message intended to warn those concerned of the existence or expected occurrence of a wind of Beaufort force 12 over a specified area.

Cf. cyclone warning, gale warning, storm warning, typhoon warning

Hydatid disease Intestinal and liver (sometimes pulmonary) infection, often clinically silent, caused by the larvae or cysts of the *Echinococcus* tapeworm, which uses sheep, cattle and especially the dog as host. The Casoni test is usually indicative.

Sn: echinococcosis, hydatidosis, hydatid cyst

Cf. enteric diseases, parasitic diseases

Hydatidosis Sn: hydatid disease

Hydrogen bomb Nuclear weapon in which the explosive power is derived from fusion which liberates energy and radiation.

Sn: H-bomb, fusion bomb, thermonuclear bomb

Cf. fusion, nuclear war, fission bomb

Hydrogeological map The synthetic map of a given territory showing the extent of its hydrological structure and characteristics, the distribution and dynamics of its underground water and useful indications regarding the evaluation and harnessing of its subterranean water resources.
Cf. water harnessing

Hydrography
1. Science that deals with the complex system of variations in the water covering the earth's surface. The instrument is the hydrograph.
2. Applied science which compiles and cartographically presents the navigable depths of the oceans and of the surrounding areas to help safe navigation.

Hydrological basin Sn: river basin

Hydrology The science that deals with the hydrosphere. Depending on the field of application, there is marine hydrology (oceanography) and continental hydrography (potamology, limnology, hydrogeology, glaciology, etc.).
Cf. hydrosphere

Hydrosphere The complex of all the waters of the globe existing between the atmosphere, the lithosphere, the continental waters, the oceans and the seas.
Cf. atmosphere

Hygiene Science that deals with the principles, methods and practical aspects of disease prevention, sanitation and improvement of health. It is usually divided into such fields as personal hygiene, domestic hygiene, food hygiene, industrial hygiene.

Hyogo World Conference on Disaster Reduction In January 2005, the WCDR at Hyogo, Japan, set important standards for the improvement of risk and disaster management. Inter alia UNISDR developed a useful basic list of disaster terminology, some reflected in this Dictionary.
Cf. ISDR, OCHA

Hypernutrition The opposite of undernutrition, resulting in a pathological state due to excessive intake of food, rich in calories, leading to obesity.
Sn: overnutrition, gluttony
Cf. malnutrition

Hypocentre
1. Ballistics: The point of the ground vertically beneath an air explosion of a nuclear bomb.
Sn: ground zero
2. Seismology: The focus of earth crust movements directly beneath the point of an earthquake.
Cf. epicentre

Hypovitaminosis Deficiency in a given vitamin, leading to disease.
Sn: vitamin deficiency

Hypoxia A fall in the physiological level of oxygen to the tissues despite adequate supply of blood, constituting a health hazard.

Hysteria A psychological disturbance with uncontrollable emotional outbursts, convulsions, anaesthesia, fear, etc. May be triggered by unusual crises, such as a disaster.

I

Iatrogenic illness Illness or accident that can be related to the actions of a physician, nurse or pharmacist or that may result from a stay in a hospital. The latter is called nosocomial illness.

Ice break-up The fall of ice walls and the disappearance of the ice cover in polar and semi-arctic regions due to climate change and hydrogeological phenomena. This is increasing due to global warming.

Ice pack The masses of ice in the polar regions formed by freezing of sea water. Examples: coastal ice pack, floating ice pack. This is decreasing due to global warming.
Sn: barrier, pack ice

Ice storm Intense formation of frost and ice on objects by the freezing of drops of rain or drizzle on impact.
Sn: glaze storm

Icterus Sn: jaundice

Identity theft A serious fraudulent act when an unauthorized person steals and transfers one's key identifying information, such as name, address, social security number, tax and bank numbers, and other personal information illegally to obtain advantages, credit or other services in the name of the victim.
Cf. hacking

Illegal immigrant An undocumented alien, who has entered a country irregularly with the aim of residing there temporarily or permanently. Asylum seekers are usually not treated as illegal immigrants.
Cf. migration, territorial asylum

Immigrant Person who arrives in a new country for personal, economic, social or political reasons and who plans to reside there.
Cf. emigrant, immigration, migrant

Immigration The massive arrival of persons in a country other than their own, usually following a disaster or political upheaval, and the process of their settling in the host country.
Cf. displaced persons, emigration, exodus, migration, refugee

Immunity Medical: The condition of being non-susceptible to an infectious disease. (Cf. immunization).
Diplomatic: The international status of being free from foreign legislation,

to cross frontiers and to carry diplomatic pouch without search or customs restrictions. (Cf. diplomatic immunity)

Immunization Rendering a person or animal immune to certain infections by the process of injecting either an antigen or a serum containing specific antibodies.
Cf. vaccination, immunity, Expanded Programme on Immunization (WHO)

Immunodeficiency Defective or deficient immunological mechanisms of the body due to insufficiency in one of the components of the immune process or to a defect in the B-lymphocyte or T-lymphocyte systems. Immunological deficit may result from infection, as AIDS, or excessive radiation, as in nuclear war, or toxic substances.
Sn: immune deficiency, immunological deficit
Cf. acquired immunodeficiency syndrome

Impact Refers to strong contact between two elements or events. The influence can be positive or negative. In disasters, it refers to the immediate damage and continuing harmful effects or results of the event. In society, a positive impact may be the effects of equitable legislation on the people.

Impairment A physical, mental or psychological deficiency in a person, or a specific organ or function, momentary or lasting, that interferes with or decreases the ability of thinking, performance or function, resulting in a handicapped, disabled or otherwise diminished person.

Impartiality Action, position or belief that makes no distinction of nationality, race, religion, colour, wealth, social condition or political conviction and in assistance applies only to the service of relief in measure of the needs of the victim's suffering – Red Cross.

Imprescriptible Right: A right that cannot be taken away or abrogated under any circumstances. Inalienable.
Cf. human rights
Crime: The absence of time limit for the investigation or sentencing of certain very serious crimes, e.g. war crimes, crimes against humanity.
Cf. impunity, transparency

Impunity The objectionable capacity of escaping legitimate punishment, or creating the conditions of avoiding and exemption from legal indictment. Corrupt persons conceiving disastrous acts or acts against humanity should be brought to justice before the International Criminal Court. The primary aim of the Rome Statutes of the International Court of Justice that came into effect on 1 July 2002 is "to put an end to impunity for the perpetrators ... of the most serious crimes". Cf. High Commissioner for Human Rights, International Criminal Court, man-conceived disaster

Incapacitating agent In chemical and biological weaponry, an agent that is intended to cause temporary disease to induce temporary mental or physical disability, the duration of which greatly exceeds the period of exposure – WHO.
Cf. lethal agent, harassing agent, chemical weapon, biological weapon

Incest Sexual abuse occurring within the family. Usually accomplished by physical force or coercion with grave psychological consequences – WGVAW.
Cf. violence against women

Incidence The number of new cases of a disease or injury or of sick persons or casualties, in a given population, in a specified period of time. It should not be confused with prevalence.
Cf. prevalence

Incident/Accident Although different in meaning and consequences, these two terms are often misused interchangeably in emergency management. Incident is a sudden, unexpected occurrence that happens by chance and is usually without very serious consequences. Accident is also a sudden, unforeseen event, but more serious, usually with some resulting damage, injury or death. Whence, accident prevention and accident department in a hospital.
Cf. accident/incident

Incident command system The aggregate of plans, procedures, equipment, human resources, communications and management operating within a unified organizational structure under responsible direction with the view to accomplishing the stated objective related to a disaster incident (ICS).
Cf. action plan

Incineration Controlled disposal of wastes by burning of domestic garbage, hospital used matter and industrial waste. Can also apply to cadavers, especially in disaster situations.

Income-based country categorization Cf. country income classification by the World Bank, 2008

Income-based mortality Poverty, riches and income differences affect peoples' health differently. Percentage of deaths in 5 main causes of disease in women aged 60 and over by country income group showed (2004), in descending order: (a) high-income developed countries: ischaemic heart disease, stroke, Alzheimer's and dementia, lower respiratory infections, lung and bronchial carcinoma; (b) middle-income countries: stroke, ischaemic heart disease, chronic obstructive pulmonary disease, hypertensive heart disease, lower respiratory infections; (c) ischaemic heart disease, stroke, lower respiratory infections, chronic obstructive pulmonary disease, diabetes mellitus – WHO.

Cf. country income classification, low-income country

Incubation period
1. The interval between the time of infection of a person or animal and the appearance of the first sign or symptom of the disease.
2. In malaria, the time needed for the completion of sporogony in the mosquito, until the stage of its becoming infective.

Cf. carrier

Indicator In management, a quantitative or qualitative benchmark or signal that shows whether an expected standard, result or impact has been attained and where corrective measures may be needed.

Indicators/Standards in disasters Cf. standards/indicators, Sphere Project

Indignez Vous!/Time for Outrage French term that can be understood as be indignant, speak out, get involved, time for outrage. A 2010 pamphlet *Indignez Vous,* under the English title of *Time for Outrage,* by Stéphane Hessel, encouraging all citizens, particularly the youth, to stand up for human rights, social values, equity and moral principles and speak out against egoism, indifference, monetarism, materialism and injustices. The term has become an internationally popular slogan for social movements, e.g. in Madrid or Cairo. The author was one of the original signatories in 1948 of the Universal Declaration of Human Rights.

Induced seismicity Earth tremors and seismic phenomena resulting from excessive man-made activity, such as atomic explosions, underground bombs, overmining, reservoir construction, oil drilling.

Industrial complex The large aggregate of physical facilities and interdependent economic activities grouped around a base industry.

Cf. rural, military-industrial complex

Inequity The opposite of equity. Inadequate services, unhygienic conditions, social inequalities, lack of access to care facilities and disdain for people's rights are not only unnecessary and avoidable in health but, in addition, are unfair, unjust and inequitable.

Cf. equity in health

Infection The entry and development or multiplication of an infectious agent (virus, bacteria, fungus, parasite) in the body of man or animal.

Cf. communicable disease, infestation, parasitic disease

Infectious disease Sn: communicable disease

Infectious hepatitis Cf. hepatitis

Infestation The penetration and development of arthropods and parasites on the body or in clothing. Cf. disinfestation, disinsection, infection, parasitic disease

Infibulation One of the three forms of female genital mutilation, consisting of the complete ablation of the clitoris, the labia minora and the labia majora at the vaginal opening. The opening is then sewn together leaving only a small passage for menstrual flow and urination.

Sn: pharaonic circumcision

Cf. female genital mutilation, FGM, female circumcision, excision, introcision

Informed consent In health care, consent must be given not only voluntarily but also such consent must be informed, the patient being well aware of what (operation, experiment, treatment or other action) he is consenting to. Special legal obligations concern the consent of (for) minors and for unconscious patients.

Cf. consent, Nuremberg Code, Helsinki Declaration

Injury Any bodily harm or organic lesion, lethal or non-lethal, caused by a mechanical, thermal, electrical, chemical or radiation agent, of such magnitude that exceeds the victim's threshold of physiological tolerance. Injury may also result from the lack of one or more vital elements, such as oxygen.

Injuries are usually classified as unintentional (e.g. traffic trauma, cuts, poisoning, fires, falls, drowning) or intentional (e.g. self-inflicted wounds, suicide, violence, fights, war injuries).

Cf. casualty, trauma, traumatic injury classification, trauma scale

Insecticide Chemical compound used for the destruction of insects harmful to man, animals and plants.

Cf. pesticide

Instant corn-soya-milk Nutritional food mixture consisting of:

59.2% cornmeal, processed, gelatinized

17.5% soya flour, defatted, toasted

15.0% non-fat dry milk, spray processed

5.5% soya oil, refined, deodorized, stabilized

2.7% mineral premix

0.1% vitamin, premix antioxidant

Sn: ICSM

Cf. food mixtures, nutrition

Insurance – disaster damage The detrimental effects of flood damage, fire or other disaster, including collateral and other unfavourable outcomes, evaluated and expressed in monetary or other terms for appropriate compensation.

Integration The unconscious processes or planned operations whereby separate elements, individuals, people or communities assemble to form a whole, in which the varying characteristics are less marked or where the resulting system acquires new characteristics.

Cf. acculturation, absorption, assimilation, minorities

Intensity (seismic) The degree of shaking or of vibrations, signifying the intensity of an earthquake as measured numerically on the Mercalli scale.

Cf. earthquake, magnitude, Mercalli scale, Richter scale

Intensive care unit A specialized medical care facility where there are physicians, surgeons, nurses, anaesthetists and other appropriate skills and the necessary equipment to provide emergency, acute and continuing care to critically ill persons.

Sn: ICU

Inter-governmental Panel on Climate Change/IPCC Established in 1988 following growing concern on the effect of human activity on climate, IPCC carries out scientific, technical and socio-economic assessments of climate change, its impact and options for mitigation. The subsequent UN Framework Convention on Climate

Change has become the principal institution on climatic issues.

Internally displaced person(s) Persons or groups of persons who have been forced or obliged to flee or to leave their homes or places of habitual residence, in particular, as a result of or in order to avoid the effects of armed conflict, situations of generalized violence, violations of human rights, or natural or man-made disasters, and who have not crossed an internationally recognized State border – UNHCR. According to established principles, these persons have the right to seek safety in another part of the country, to leave their country, to seek asylum in another country and the right to be protected against forcible return or unsafe resettlement. But these are not refugees in the juridical sense.
Cf. displaced person, refugee, IDP

International assistance Assistance provided by one or more countries or international or voluntary organizations to a country in need, usually for development or for an emergency. The four main elements of assistance within the international community are as follows:
a. The intergovernmental agencies – United Nations, European Union
b. Non-governmental organizations
c. The Red Cross
d. Bilateral agreements
Cf. bilateral cooperation, donor, non-governmental organizations, Red Cross, technical assistance

International Association for Humanitarian Medicine Brock Chisholm/IAHM A professional, non-profit, non-governmental organization that promotes and delivers health care on the principles of humanitarian medicine and named after Dr. Brock Chisholm, the first Director-General of the World Health Organization. In particular, it provides medical, surgical, nursing and rehabilitative care to patients in or from developing countries deficient in the necessary specialized expertise; brings relief to victims of disasters where health aid is lacking; mobilizes hospitals and health specialists in developed countries to receive and treat such patients free of charge; promotes the concept of health as a human right and bridge to peace and advocates humanitarian law and humanitarian principles in the practice of medicine.
Cf. humanitarian medicine, human rights, disasters, non-governmental organization, World Health Organization, World Open Hospitals

International Atomic Energy Agency/ IAEA
UN specialized agency for the peaceful uses of atomic energy; promotes the contribution of this energy to peace, health and prosperity and ensures that it is not used for military purposes.
Supervises the safety and monitors accidents of nuclear installations, but is not involved in non-peaceful nuclear (weapons) questions. Was awarded the Nobel Peace Prize.
Cf. Chernobyl, environmental pollution, nuclear reactor, transboundary pollution, United Nations, INES

International Bank for Reconstruction Cf. World Bank

International Bill of Human Rights High international legislation concerning human rights, composed of:
1. The Universal Declaration of Human Rights

2. International Covenant on Economic, Social and Cultural Rights
3. International Covenant on Civil and Political Rights
4. The Optional Protocol to the International Covenant on Civil and Political Rights – UN.

International Centre Ettore Majorana for World Laboratory of Scientific Culture Important centre in Erice, Sicily, that promotes and organizes scientific discussion, cultural activities and research into fundamental questions on humanity and society.

International Centre for Migration and Health/ICMH A non-profit organization involved in all humanitarian, educational and operational aspects of migration, population movement and welfare and health-related problems of people displaced by disasters.
Cf. migration, refugees

International Civil Defence Organization/ICDO Inter-governmental organization for society's response to serious emergencies. It develops, strengthens and coordinates civil protection for all people in different countries, collaborates with governments and other organizations in preparedness and response to natural and man-made disasters and promotes safer environment conducive to development.
Cf. civil defence, civil protection

International Committee of the Red Cross Sn: ICRC
Cf. Red Cross, International Humanitarian Law

International community A poorly defined popular term in international relations that, on the world scene,
loosely refers to the aggregate of the different governments, populations, cultures and groupings that share a commonalty in a multinational globalized world.
At a local scene, e.g. in the international city of Geneva, it refers to the varied population of diplomats and their families, foreign missions, the UN agencies and their staffs, non-governmental organizations, international schools, multinational companies and others in international activity.
Cf. community

International crimes Cf. Nuremberg Charter

International Criminal Court/ICC A permanent international tribunal based in the Hague, established in 1998 by the United Nations but independent of it, with jurisdiction on only "the most serious crimes of concern to the international community as a whole" and complementary to national criminal jurisdiction. Crimes within its jurisdiction include crimes against humanity, genocide, war crimes.
Includes the War Crimes Tribunal for the former Yugoslavia (1993), the International Criminal Tribunal for Rwanda (1994).
Cf. crimes against humanity, crime of aggression, genocide, human rights, Universal Declaration of Human Rights, war crimes, International Humanitarian Law, Nuremberg Charter

International Criminal Tribunal(s) The Security Council has established Criminal Tribunals for specific serious breaches of International Humanitarian Law.
In 1993, the ICT for the former Yugoslavia was established to prosecute

such violators in the former Yugoslavia since 1991.

In 1994, the ICT for Rwanda was mandated to prosecute perpetrators of genocide in that country.

The first ever conviction for genocide by an international court was handed down in 1998 by the ICT Rwanda in Arusha.

Cf. genocide, crimes against humanity, International Court of Justice, Nuremberg Charter of 1945

International Criminal Tribunal for Rwanda/ICTR In 1994, the UN Security Council established the ICTR at the request of Rwanda to identify and prosecute persons responsible for genocide and other violations of International Humanitarian Law during the Tutsi-Rwandan conflict.

Cf. TRC, compare with the Truth and Reconciliation Commission, genocide, IHL

International Federation of Health and Human Rights Organizations IFHHRO brings together individual and organized health workers with other rights workers for the realization of a rights-based healthy atmosphere for everyone. It recalls the responsibility of governments to reduce health and rights inequalities.

International Federation of Medical Students' Associations/IFMSA Independent federation of national medical students' organizations which, besides being concerned with standards of medical education, public health and relevant medical curricula, promotes prevention of nuclear war, training in disaster medicine and programmes for refugee health. NGO in official relations with WHO and the UN system.

International Federation of Red Cross and Red Crescent Societies Sn: IFRC (Federation, previously League)

Cf. Red Cross

International Federation of Surgical Colleges/IFSC The senior surgical confederation in the world that promotes the attainment of the highest standards in surgery, teaching, ethics and surgical practice worldwide; assists developing and emerging countries in raising their professional standards and encourages essential surgery within the WHO concept of primary health care. Advisor to the World Health Organization and to ECOSOC on all matters surgical.

Cf. World Health Organization

International health Study and systematic comparison of the multiple and variable factors that influence the health of human populations in different countries, the transmission of disease across boundaries and the resulting regulations and measures that need to be taken for improvement of global health.

Cf. global health, epidemiology, International Health Regulations, World Health Organization

International Health Regulations/ IHR A set of globally applied rules, revised and updated in 2005 by the World Health Assembly, concerning national and international health. The purpose and scope of the Regulations are "to prevent, protect against, control and provide a public health response to the international spread of disease in ways that are commensurate with and restricted to public health risks, and which avoid unnecessary interference with international traffic and trade" – IHR.

Cf. World Health Organization, international health, global health, quarantine

International Humanitarian Law/ IHL Humanitarian legislation comprised mainly of the four Geneva Conventions (1949) and its two additional protocols (1977), intimately associated with the responsibilities of the International Committee of the Red Cross and the National Red Cross or Red Crescent Societies. Its main purpose is to provide a codified set of rules for the protection and assistance to victims of armed conflict. Also referred to as the Law of War, the Law of Geneva.
Cf. Geneva Conventions, humanitarian, Red Cross

International Labour Organization/ ILO UN agency of tripartite composition representing governments, employers and workers; ILO is concerned with setting and monitoring labour standards within economic and social development, promoting better working conditions and employment opportunities, with particular care to occupational health and human rights.

International law The corpus of principles, rules, treaties and procedures that govern the conduct, relationships and exchanges between and among States and juridical institutions. Laws that concern health include, *inter alia*, the International Health Regulations, the Geneva Protocols, human rights laws, environmental and climate laws, International Humanitarian Laws, relevant UN protocols.

International Medical Products Anti-Counterfeiting Task Force Counterfeit drugs and unapproved medicines have become a very large illegal business that not only deters from effective medication but also constitutes health hazards. IMPACT is a task force for the detection and suppression of such practices.
Cf. Medicines transparency alliance

International Monetary Fund/ IMF United Nations agency that promotes international financial cooperation, facilitates trade and stability, helps poor nations meet their programmes and assists in financial crises. IMF

International Nuclear Event Scale/ INES A 7-level logarithmic scale introduced in 1990 by the International Atomic Energy Agency (IAEA) to describe the comparative magnitude of a nuclear event. It comprises 4 accident and 3 incident levels, as follows: 7 – major accident, 6 – serious accident, 5 – accident with wider, off-site consequences, 4 – accident with local consequences; 3 – serious incident, 2 – incident, 1 – anomaly, 0 – deviation, without safety implications. The Chernobyl disaster (1986) was of level 7; Mayak accident (1957) level 6; Three Mile Island (1979) level 5; Sellafield (1955) level 4; Sellafield (2005) level 3; Forsmark (2006) level 2; Gravelines (2009) level 1; Hyderabad (2002) level 0.
Cf. International Atomic Energy Agency, nuclear disaster, accident, incident

International Organization for Migration/IOM Founded in response to massive migrations after World War II, IOM is the principal intergovernmental organization involved in all issues of migration management, policies, health, facilitation and regulation.
Cf. migration, emigration

International Physicians for the Prevention of Nuclear War/ IPPNW International non-governmental association of physicians that strives to mobilize the moral and social responsibility of the medical profession in face of nuclear war and encourages actions and decisions for the prevention of nuclear war. Received the Nobel Peace Prize.
Sn: IPPNW
Cf. nuclear war, GLAWARS Report, WHOPAX Report

International Programme on Chemical Safety/IPCS A United Nations initiative, IPCS is managed jointly by the World Health Organization, the UN Environment Programme and the International Labour Organization, with the aim of providing an internationally evaluated scientific basis on which countries may develop their own chemical safety measures, to strengthen national capabilities for prevention and treatment of harmful effects of chemicals and to manage the health aspects of chemical emergencies. It runs the INTOX network which facilitates rapid toxicological information among some 120 centres.
Cf. chemical accident, environmental disaster, Bhopal, Seveso, UN hazard classification

International protection Protection of refugees undertaken by the High Commissioner for Refugees on behalf of the international community.
Cf. refugee protection, UNHCR

International Recovery Platform Forum created following the Hyogo Framework for Action to facilitate the integration of risk reduction factors in post-disaster recovery operations.

International Rehabilitation Council for Torture Victims/IRCT An independent, international health professional organization that promotes and supports the rehabilitation of torture victims, works for the prevention of torture worldwide and teaches values and accepts shared responsibility for the eradication of torture. Publishes the journal Torture.
Cf. torture, Universal Declaration of Human Rights

International Social EMS In French, SAMU Social International, institution that aims (a) to provide emergency social assistance in insalubrious big cities to all who are homeless, lonely, hungry, friendless or in other mental or physical distress and (b) to promote and establish similar comprehension, facilities, institutions and resources for emergency social assistance in all urban centres worldwide – Emmanuelli.

International Strategy for Disaster Reduction/ISDR The United Nations designated the years 1990–1999 as the International Decade for Natural Disaster Reduction (IDNDR), when extensive studies and action were carried out in all aspects of disasters. At the completion of the decade, from 2000 onwards, the programme continues as the UN International Strategy for Disaster Reduction (ISDR), through OCHA, the UN Office for the Coordination of Humanitarian Affairs.
Cf. disaster, disaster management, United Nations, OCHA

International Telecommunication Union/ITU UN specialized agency for international cooperation in the rational use and improvement of all

telecommunications, including radio, television, Internet, telegraph, telephone and satellite space communications. Important activity in early warning systems for disasters.
Cf. satellite, space station

International traffic For the purposes of the International Health Regulations, the term means "the movement of persons, baggage, cargo, containers, conveyances, goods or postal parcels across an international border, including international trade". These may be subject to inspection to determine if a public health risk exists.

International treaty/Treaty Agreement formally ratified between States, or between States and international organizations, aiming at establishing international order in a specific domain. Treaty is one of the instruments that confer legal status to the rights and obligations of the signatory States.
Cf. treaty, convention, protocol, declaration, charter

Interpol Full name: International Criminal Police Organization (ICPO), founded in 1923, with the purpose of mutual assistance between and among the law enforcing authorities of all the different states across boundaries in the suppression of ordinary law crimes and coordination and documentation regarding international crime.

Intertidal The coastal strip between the highest and the lowest levels of the tide.
Cf. tide

Intertropical convergence zone An atmospheric area above the Atlantic ocean roughly midway between South America (Brazil) and Africa (Senegal) where strong meteorological turbulences are common, with very high winds, storms and lightning that can cause aeronautical disturbances. The most catastrophic event was on 1 June 2009, resulting in the disappearance of a civilian aircraft with the death of all 228 passengers and crew, without aerial warning. Sometimes referred to as the Bermuda Triangle

Intestinal diseases Sn: enteric diseases
Cf. diarrhoeal diseases

Intifada Arabic word approximately meaning uprising. The Palestinian freedom uprising against Israeli forces, mainly in 1987–1993, repeated over several years.
Cf. guerrilla

INTOX network A programme of the IPCS that links about 120 centres in some 70 countries for rapid electronic access to toxicological, analytical and clinical expertise on dangerous and military chemical agents.
Cf. International Programme on Chemical Safety, chemical weapons

Intrauterine device/IUD A small medical device inserted into the uterus for contraception.

Introcision Widening of the vaginal opening by tearing it downwards using three fingers bound with string.
Cf. female genital mutilation, female circumcision, excision, infibulation

Inviolability That cannot be violated, transgressed, infringed. Inviolability refers to three notions: (a) the fundamental human rights that are inalienable and cannot be violated under any circumstances, (b) personal inviolability of a diplomat or diplomatic courier, making it impossible and illegal to be submitted to any form of arrest or detention and (c) inviolability of the premises of an embassy or mission or of a diplomatic pouch.

Iodine An essential micronutrient and important for normal basal metabolism. Its deficiency results in goitre. Used also prophylactically against nuclear radioactivity.

Cf. Lugol's iodine, goitre, thyroid, nuclear accident

Iodine-131 Radioactive iodine. Following a nuclear accident or atomic explosion, the released radioactive isotope risks to be absorbed by the thyroid, or be dissolved in water, with serious biological consequences in man. The administration of stable iodine can prevent such absorption and is used prophylactically.

Cf. Lugol's iodine, iodine

Ion An originally neutral atom which has become electrically charged by losing or acquiring electrons. Loss of an electron results in a positive ion (cation) and acquisition in a negative ion (anion).

Cf. ionizing radiation, ionosphere

Ionizing radiation Any electromagnetic radiation that, when passing through matter, can produce ions. Includes X-rays, alpha-beta-gamma rays, neutrons, protons.

Cf. ion, cosmic radiation, radiation injury, kerma

Ionosphere The zone of the atmosphere, from about 70 km to 500 km, in which charged particles, ions and electrons are formed by photoionization under the effect of the sun's radiation.

Ionospheric sounding Determination of the vertical profile of the electronic density of the ionosphere, by measuring the echo of multiple frequency radio-electric signals.

Cf. ionosphere, meteorological sounding, sounding

Irrigation In agriculture, the watering of land to compensate for a lack or shortage of rainfall in certain areas and periods.

Isobar On a map or chart, the line drawn joining the points that have equal barometric pressure.

Isohyet On a map or chart, the line drawn joining the points that have equal amounts of precipitation.

Isotherm On a map or chart, the line drawn joining the points that have the same temperature.

Isotope Each of the nuclides having the same atomic number (electrons) and thus sharing identical chemical properties. (The number of neutrons differs.)

Istituto Nazionale sui Diritti dell'Uomo International Institute on Human Rights, situated in Trieste, Italy, for study, research and promotion of human rights. Associated with the Council of Europe.

Cf. human rights

J

Japan Medical Team for Disaster Relief/JMTDR Supported by the medical profession and the Japan International Cooperation Agency (JICA), JMTDR is a major organization providing emergency medical response worldwide as well as studying and advising on disaster management problems.

Cf. Asia-Pacific Conferences on Disaster Medicine, international assistance

Jaundice A yellow discolouration of the skin, the sclera of the eyes and other tissues due to excess bile in the circulation. May be caused by several diseases, including hepatitis, malaria, haemorrhagic fever, yellow fever, wrong blood transfusion, haemolysis, drugs.

Sn: icterus

Cf. hepatitis, yellow fever

Jettison In transport and shipping, it means washing overboard. Voluntary throwing of cargo overboard in emergencies to prevent further damage to the ship or to other cargo. In cases of general average, the value of jettisoned goods enters into the calculation of expenses.

Cf. average

Jihad Arabic term for a holy war undertaken by Muslims against unbelievers. Literally means "effort" in Muslim struggle on behalf of God and Islam.

Johannesburg Summit World Summit conference held in Johannesburg, South Africa, in 2002, consecrated to sustainable development.

Jus cogens Latin legal term indicating customary law and its validity according to the Vienna Convention of 1969.

K

K-2 Mix High-protein food mixture containing casein hydrolysate, sucrose and milk.

Cf. food mixtures

Kala-azar Sn: visceral leishmaniasis

Kamikaze Japanese word for suicide bomber. An attack in which, for idealistic, military or other reasons, the attacker plans or accepts to die in the process of his/her suicidal attack.

Sn: suicide bomber

Cf. suicide attack, self-molestation

Kerma Acronym for Kinetic Energy Released in Matter, the measure of intensity of ionizing radiation at a given place. The dose is expressed in grays (Gy).

Cf. ionizing radiation

Kidnapping Abduction, forced disappearance or unlawful carrying away of a child or other person to use as hostage, for gain, political pressure, torture or any other purpose. From kid=child, nap=to steal.

Cf. abduction, disappearance

Kiloton A measure of the explosive power of nuclear arms, equivalent to 1,000 tons of TNT. The bomb on Hiroshima was of 12.5 kt, on Nagasaki 22 kt.

Sm: kt

Cf. megaton, nuclear war, TNT

Kimberley Process Kimberley Process Certification Scheme to control the rough diamond trade.

Cf. blood diamonds, conflict diamonds, kleptocracy

Kleptocracy Literally, government by thieves. The unethical and illegal practice of certain presidents, rulers and autocrats to amass and store in secret accounts and foreign properties enormous personal wealth derived from illicit appropriations, corruption, coercion, threats and occult stealing (klepto) from the nation's treasury and citizens' taxes, often leaving their own country in poverty. President Mobutu of Zaire, Marcos of the Philippines, Duvalier of Haiti, Sani Abacha of Nigeria, Suharto of Indonesia and Gaddafi of Libya are recent examples of the many kleptocrats.

Cf man-conceived disaster, corruption, blood diamonds

Knowledge translation The exchange, synthesis and ethically-sound application of knowledge within a complex of interactions among researchers and users to accelerate the capture of the benefits of research for the people through improved health, more effective services and products, and a strengthened health care system – CIHR.

Kobe earthquake Cf. Great Hanshin earthquake of 1995

Kosher Hebrew word for food that is fit to eat and conforms to Jewish religious prescriptions.
Cf. custom, halal

Kwashiorkor A serious form of protein-calorie malnutrition that occurs most frequently in infants and young children about the time of weaning. Presents with oedema, wasting, dermatitis, hair changes, anaemia, diarrhoea, lethargy, apathy and stunted growth.
Cf. anaemia, malnutrition, protein-calorie malnutrition, marasmus

Kyoto   Protocol United   Nations Framework on Climate Change, undertaken in 1997 in Kyoto, Japan, calling on all countries, particularly the industrialized states, to reduce their emissions of gases that cause global warming (CO_2, CFC, methane, etc.) by 5.2% by the years 2008–2012 in relation to the 1990 levels. Ratified in 2005.
Cf. glasshouse effect, global warming, chlorofluorocarbons, ozone depletion, atmospheric pollution

L

Laerdal pocket mask A folding pocket mask with oxygen insufflation nipple for assisted mouth-to-mouth ventilation, applied to the injured in emergencies by trained personnel.

La Hague Town in Northern France, site of an important nuclear waste processing plant. (Do not confuse with the Hague in the Netherlands). Receives uranium, plutonium, nuclear spent material and reprocesses them, sending the extracted product to other plants and the mud débris for disposal. Much controversy surrounds these dangerous operations and nuclear waste.
Cf. Sellafield, nuclear wastes

Lahar Acid ash flow, generally enrobing volcanic blocks as a result of imbibition of the ash with water.
Cf. ash flow, volcano

Landmine Treaty Cf. Ottawa Convention, ICBL

Landmines Sn: antipersonnel mines
Cf. mines, Ottawa Convention, ICBL, Cranfield Mine Action

Landslide A massive and more or less rapid sliding down of soil and rock, causing damage in its path.
Cf. avalanche, mudslide

La Niňa The opposite of El Niňo.
Cf. El Niňo

Laser Acronymic name for "light amplification by stimulated emission of radiation", a device that uses focused light beams to provide powerful directed force for a wide variety of applications, from medical therapeutic instruments, sophisticated machinery, to lethal beams and weaponry.

Lassa fever A viral disease of wild rodents, highly contagious and fatal to man. Sporadic cases of outbreaks occur mainly in West Africa.
Cf. haemorrhagic fever

Latitude In the geographical system of spherical coordinates, the angular distance of point from a fundamental plane, computed from this plane 0–90° towards the (positive) North Pole and 0 to −90° towards the South. The equator marks 0°.
Cf. geographic longitude

Latrine A simple toilet facility dug in the ground for the disposal of human excreta, to minimize spread of disease and contamination of the water and environment. Various forms are used in disaster situations and refugee communities. Some types are deep trench latrines, bore hole, shallow, straddle and bucket latrines. The Oxfam emergency sanitation unit is a good model.
Cf. chlorine, environmental hygiene

Lava flow The residual molten magma and ash that, after a volcanic eruption, flows down rather slowly over the mountain side.

Law of Geneva Cf. law of war, International Humanitarian Law

Law of the sea The system of international laws and regulations governing the marine areas and their utilization and the persons associated with such activity.

Law of War The law of armed conflict, the corpus of rules which in wartime prescribe and limit methods and means of warfare, protect the health providers in the field and spare from attacks the persons who are not, or no longer, participating in hostilities. These are codified in the 1949 Geneva Conventions and the 1977 Additional Protocols.
Sn: International Humanitarian Law, law of Geneva
Cf. International Committee of the Red Cross, Geneva Conventions, crimes against humanity, International Criminal Court

Lawfare A new term denoting the manipulation or exploitation of the international legal system with the veiled purpose of supplementing military and political objectives of aggression or aggressive war.
Cf. warfare

LD50 Lethal dose 50. The amount of a toxic substance or of radiation that is needed to kill 50% of the persons in a population in a given time.
Cf. dose, lethal dose 50

Lead time The length of time elapsed between the announcement of a particular hazard and its arrival.
Also used for the time allowed between a disaster and mobilization of resources against it

Least developed countries/LDC A category of States that according to United Nations, criteria are deemed structurally handicapped in their development process and in need of the highest degree of attention from the international community for development. ECOSOC uses three criteria for this categorization: (a) low income, GDP per capita under $900; (b) human resources: low index of nutrition, health, education and adult literacy; (c) economic vulnerability: instability of agriculture, exports of goods and services, non-traditional activities, merchandise exports and handicap of economic smallness. LDCs constitute 49 States, 10.7% of the world population and 0.5% of the world GNP – UNCTAD, 2001.
Term less and less used; prefer low-income country.
Cf. developing countries, low-income countries, Millennium Development Goals, G-20

Legionnaire's disease A form of bronchopneumonia caused by the *Legionella pneumophila*, transmitted man to man and in steamy and moist conditions, as through air-conditioning ducts.

Leishmaniasis An infectious group of protozoan diseases caused by Leishmania and transmitted by the sandfly.

Cf. cutaneous leishmaniasis, kala-azar, visceral leishmaniasis, neglected tropical disease

Leptospirosis An infectious and potentially serious disease (with meningitis, liver failure) caused by a variety of Leptospira, transmitted from animals through contaminated water, vegetation and food. Can cause jaundice (Weil's syndrome). Heavy floods in 1988 caused an epidemic of leptospirosis in Brazil.
Sn: Weil's disease, infectious jaundice
Cf. epidemic, jaundice, zoonosis

Lethal agent A chemical or biological weapon that is intended to cause death when man is exposed to concentrations well within the capability of delivery for military purposes – WHO.
Cf. incapacitating agent, harassing agent

Lethal dose 50 The radiation dose that kills 50% of the exposed people in a given time.
Sn: LD50

Levee Water-retaining earthwork along a river or coastline to prevent flooding from waves or tides.
Sn: dike, embankment, bank, bund

Life expectancy The probability of the average duration of life in a community, statistically based on death rates.
Cf. death rate, mortality rate

Life support Emergency: Immediate help, specialized techniques and apparatus applied in assisting a seriously injured person or a disaster victim to maintain the vital functions.
Sn: cardiopulmonary resuscitation, CPR
Global: The Earth's naturally balanced ecosystem necessary to maintain human life.
Cf. ecosystem

Lifelines The community facilities and public systems, such as potable water, sanitation, energy, shelter, transport and communications, that ensure the basic life support services, especially in emergencies.
Cf. primary health care, survival chain

Lighter Barge that comes alongside a vessel on which cargo is unloaded or loaded, when this cannot be done at a quay or wharf.

Littoral Coastline where the sea, land and atmosphere meet.
Sn: coast

Livelihood The general capacity of sustenance and living. The World Food Programme defines it as a person's or community's capabilities, assets and activities that are required to ensure a means of living.
Cf. sustainable livelihood, development, World Food Programme, hunger

Lixiviation Degradation of the soil or of certain superficial layers by the downward flow of earth mixtures in solution.

Logistics The strategies and range of operations concerned with supply, storage, handling, distribution, transport and evacuation of material and people.

Longitudinal study Prospective study. Study of a population over a period of time starting with the present.

Louse infestation Skin condition caused by the invasion of the body by lice. Can lead to secondary infection.
Sn: pediculosis

Low birth weight A baby weighing less than 2,500 g (5 pounds 82 ounces) at birth. Very low birth weight: less than 1,500 g.

Low-income/Lower-middle-income countries The World Bank categorizes (2008) according to Gross National Income (GNI, previously GNP): low-income country: US$975 or less; low-middle income country: US$976–3,855.
Cf. upper middle income, high income, country income categorization, developing country, least developed country

Lugol's iodine A pharmaceutical solution of iodine and potassium iodide. Its ingestion saturates the thyroid gland which takes up the iodine in the blood, a property that is used as a prophylactic measure in exposure to radioactivity, and its administration blocks further iodine uptake by the thyroid.
Sn: Lugol's solution
Cf. basal metabolic rate, goitre, iodine, thyroid

Lymphatic filariasis A debilitating and stigmatizing disease due to worm infection that blocks the lymphatic circulation.
Sn: elephantiasis

M

Macroclimate The general large-scale climate covering a wide area or country, as distinguished from mesoclimate and microclimate that cover smaller, even specific areas.
Cf. climate

Macronutrient/Micronutrient Cf. nutrients

Mad cow disease An infectious brain damage in the cow believed to be caused by a new class of infective agents, called prions. Can be transmitted to other animals and man, causing visual disturbances, neuromuscular disequilibrium and inevitable death. Can spread in epidemic proportions among animals and men over several years. The human variant is called Creutzfeldt-Jakob disease.
Sn: bovine spongiform encephalopathy, BSE
Cf. Creutzfeldt-Jakob disease, zoonosis

Mafia Organized, secret, criminal association of wrongdoing persons carrying out illegal acts, violence, blackmail, murder, kidnapping, etc., with the view to group or personal gains and enrichment.
Cf. Palermo Convention Against Organized Crime, narcotraffic

Magma The molten stratum beneath the earth's crust.

Magnetic storm Unforeseen and sudden storm with a variation of the declination by up to 2–3° in a few hours and lasting for several days.

Magnitude of earthquake The "size" of an earthquake, expressing the amount of energy released in the form of elastic waves as measured by a seismograph, on a scale such as Richter's.
Cf. earthquake, intensity, Mercalli scale, Richter scale

Major accident hazard A chemical, biological or radioactive substance that has the potential of giving rise to a major accident or disaster. The subject of the European Directive 501/82 and of the UN class of hazardous substances.
Cf. chemical accident, hazard, Seveso, UN hazard classification, IPCS

Major hazard installation A stockpile or store of large quantities of dangerous, hazardous substances and energy in one place, e.g. refineries, petrochemical plants, chemical production factories, LPG stores, water treatment plants – ILO.

Cf. major accident hazard, major technological accident

Major technological accident Serious technological emergency, such as a major emission, fire or explosion resulting from uncontrolled developments in the course of an industrial activity, leading to serious danger to man, immediate or delayed, inside or outside the establishment, and to the environment and involving one or more dangerous substances – ILO.
Cf. major accident hazard, major hazard installation, technological disaster

Malabsorption syndrome A malnutritional condition, mainly in children, with defective absorption of fluids and other nutritive substances, presenting with weakness, wasting, fatty diarrhoea, anaemia and neurological disorders.
Sn: sprue, tropical sprue
Cf. kwashiorkor

Malaria A parasitic infection characterized by cycles of chills, fever, sweating, anaemia, enlarged spleen and chronic relapsing course. Four types of parasites – *plasmodium vivax, P. falciparum, P. malariae* and *P. ovale* – affect man, through infection by the anopheles mosquito. Most malarious areas are in the tropics. Disasters, like floods and refugee encampments, and poor environments are conducive to the propagation of the disease.
Cf. endemic, parasitic diseases

Malaria, uncomplicated Uncomplicated malaria is defined as asymptomatic malaria without signs of severity or clinical or laboratory evidence of vital organ dysfunction. The signs and symptoms are non-specific, and malaria is suspected clinically mostly on the basis of fever or a history of fever – WHO.
Cf. malaria

Malnutrition A general or specific pathological state, resulting from an absence or deficiency in the diet of one or more essential nutriments, and either clinically manifest or detectable only by examination or physiological tests. Malnutrition can also be due to an excess of the wrong food.
Cf. nutritional deficiency, kwashiorkor, protein-calorie malnutrition, undernutrition

Managed care A system of providing health care in which the providers do not receive direct reimbursement for their specific services, instead, they work for a fixed sum of money to cover the costs of care of each patient. This, mainly American system, is expected to encourage resource savings and diminish health-care costs.
Cf. health promotion

Management Cf. disaster management, emergency management

Man-conceived disaster Distinct from a man-made disaster, man-conceived refers to disastrous actions like genocide, death camps, ethnic cleansing, forced disappearance, pauperization, torture and other acts against humanity that are obscenely conceived, cold-bloodedly planned and indecently perpetrated with impunity by evil rulers, dictators or kleptocrats with the aim of inflicting maximum suffering, death and destruction, in full violation of personal, social and cultural rights of humanity. While the response to man-made disasters is scientific, humanitarian and managerial, the response to man-conceived disasters must be through the International Criminal Court – Gunn.

Cf. crimes against humanity, deportation, ethnic cleansing, forced disappearance, genocide, human rights, International Criminal Court, impunity, kleptocracy, mafia, man-made disaster, torture, Universal Declaration of Human Rights

Mandate Power or authorization given by a superior authority, legal body or international institution to another party to execute, supervise or control specified functions.

Mandate refugee Person who is considered to be a refugee according to the criteria of the statutes of the United Nations High Commissioner for Refugees.
Cf. refugee, UNHCR

Manifest In transport and shipping, list of the consignments placed on board an aircraft or ship.

Manioc Meal made from the roots of the cassava plant. The staple food in many tropical countries.
Cf. cassava, staple food

Man-made disaster A disaster caused not by natural phenomena but by human or society's action, involuntary or voluntary, sudden or slow, directly or indirectly, with grave consequences to the population and the environment. Examples: technological disaster, toxicological disaster, desertification, environmental pollution, conflicts, epidemics, fires.
Sn: human-made disaster
Cf. disaster, natural disaster, technological disaster, man-conceived disaster

Mantoux test A skin test using tuberculin to show whether a person has or has had infection with the tuberculosis bacillus.
Cf. tuberculosis

Marasmus Cf. nutritional marasmus

Marburg disease A highly lethal disease prevalent in Central Africa, caused by a filovirus. Also in epidemic form.
Sn: African haemorrhagic fever

Marginality The position of an individual or group of persons who stand on the boundary between two groups, feeling marginalized and uncertain about their status in either.
Cf. absorption, acculturation, ethnic group, minorities, discrimination

Maritime climate The climate of the regions adjacent to the sea, characterized by small diurnal or annual (or both) amplitudes of temperature and by high relative humidity.
Cf. continental climate, equatorial climate, monsoon climate, mountain climate, tropical climate

Mass casualty situation In an emergency or disaster with a great number of victims or injured, a situation where their numbers and needs far outweigh the ability of the existing system to handle, where the demand for medical care is greater than the facilities available. In a mass casualty situation, the capacity of a hospital is considered to be its ability to manage a load of patients approximately in the range of 20% of its normal bed capacity.

MAST Acronymic name for military antishock trousers, also known as PASG, pneumatic antishock garment. A double-layer pneumatic suit inflated with a foot or bicycle-pump and used for a patient in shock. The principle is to raise the blood pressure, control bleeding and promote haemostasis in emergency situations. It is now being used less frequently as it is not free from complications.
Cf. emergency medical services, first aid

Maximum acceptable concentration The presence of a pollutant or potentially harmful agent in the air, in food, in water to a degree that, on absorption by an organism, it will remain below the maximum allowed dose.
Cf. absorbed dose, maximum acceptable dose

Maximum acceptable dose The maximum quantity of a substance or energy which, in the present state of scientific knowledge, does not seem to provoke appreciable disturbances in the receiving person or his descendants.
Cf. absorbed dose, maximum acceptable concentration, nuclear energy

Mayak nuclear accident A town in Russia, site of the Kyshtym military nuclear reactor where, on 29 September 1957, the cooling system failed, causing a steam explosion releasing 70–80 tons of radioactive material into the atmosphere; rated as serious accident level 6 on the INES scale.
Cf. Chernobyl, Three Mile Island, nuclear accident, fallout, Fukushima, International Nuclear Event Scale

Measles A highly contagious acute disease of childhood, characterized by a spreading skin rash, fever, cough, coryza, conjunctivitis, eruption of the buccal mucosa (Koplik's spots) and prostration. Overcrowding and disaster conditions are conducive to outbreaks, with high mortality, especially among the malnourished.
Cf. Expanded Programme on Immunization

Measures of effectiveness/MOE In assessment techniques, the qualitative and quantitative criteria used to predict or correlate the value or measure of an organization or a system, such as disaster management. Such measures must be appropriate, quantifiable, sensitive, timely, cost-effective and meaningful – Burkle.
Cf. disaster management, damage probability

Médecins sans Frontières (MSF) Doctors without Borders. Important and efficient international organization originally started in France, to provide medical assistance in disasters and conflicts, even when claims of State sovereignty put difficulties for their humanitarian work. MSF's acknowledged and persistent action spearheaded the "right to intervene" concept, and its continuous humanitarian services won it the Nobel Peace Prize, 1999. Colloquially also referred to as "French Doctors".
Cf. international assistance, humanitarian medicine, right to intervene

Media factor Cf. CNN effect

Medicaid The American programme that provides "safety net" health-care coverage to the poor and disadvantaged people in the United States.
Cf. Medicare, national health system

Medical act Any intervention or effort by a medically qualified person to bring health assistance to a patient.
In health economics, it is the measurement unit for calculating health-care costs, health expenditure and for quantifying a health professional's remuneration.
Cf. managed care

Medical audit A thorough examination and evaluation by qualified persons of a selection of representative medical records of a health establishment with the view to assessing the quality of its health care.

Medical care quality The degree to which health services for individuals and for populations increase the likelihood of desired health outcomes and are consistent with current professional knowledge – Inst. Med. US.

The three main elements of quality are structure, process and outcomes.

Medical tourism Travel by a patient across international borders for the express purpose of seeking and receiving medical or surgical care.

Medicare In the predominantly private-liberal system of health care in America, a system of health service for people over age 65. Funded and administered by the Federal Government.

Cf. Medicaid, national health service

Medicines Transparency Alliance An organization that, within the spirit of good governance for medical programmes, focuses on affordability and availability of good quality medicaments through country-led actions that promote efficiency in the drug purchasing chain, notably through transparency and accountability.

Cf. essential drugs

Medicus Mundi Humanitarian organization that carries out important studies, research, publications and field work on the health of disfavoured populations and developing countries.

Mediterranean Council for Burns and Fire Disasters (MBC) Started by surgical burn specialists to raise regional standards and improve response to burns and fires, the organization has grown in its field of action and geographically. Designated by the World Health Organization as scientific Collaborating Centre on Burns and Fire Disasters and by the United Nations Economic and Social Council as a specialized NGO, it has pioneered links between burns as a clinical problem and fires as a societal disaster management problem. It carries out research, studies, prevention, emergency missions and helps developing countries in these fields. Now expanded as the Euro-Mediterranean Council. It has close ties with the International Association for Humanitarian Medicine Brock Chisholm.

Cf. burn, fire disaster, International Association for Humanitarian Medicine, United Nations, MBC

MEDLARS/MEDLINE Acronymic name for Medical Literature Analysis and Retrieval System, superseded by Medline, the US National Library of Medicine's extensive international computerized online system for international and systematic medical literature search.

Mefloquine A quinine derivative medicament used against malaria when there is chloroquine resistance.

Cf. chloroquine, malaria

Megatonnage equivalent A measure of the explosive power of nuclear arms, equivalent to 4.187×10^{15} J, or about the equivalent of one million tons of TNT.

Sm: Mt, MTE5

Cf. fission bomb, fusion bomb, nuclear war, kiloton

Melamine A chemical used extensively for dishware and kitchenware that leaves traces in food. No health problems in normal use but toxic at high levels. The Codex allows max.2.5 mg/kg in animal feed.

Meltdown A major disastrous event in a nuclear facility caused by the over-

heating of the nuclear rods in the reactor.
Cf. Chernobyl, Three Mile Island, Fukushima

Meneghetti Foundation The Antonio Meneghetti Foundation encourages, finances and awards scholarships for scientific, humanistic and international developmental endeavours based on an ontological interpretation of ethics and human values.

Mercalli scale Numerical scale from 1 to 12, indicating the intensity of an earthquake:

1. No movement felt
2. Felt by a few people
3. Felt indoors, slight swaying of hanging objects
4. Vibration felt, squeaking of wooden buildings
5. Felt by almost everyone, awakening from sleep
6. Felt by everyone, fright and flight
7. Difficulty to stand up, objects and chimneys fall
8. Driving difficult, partial collapse of buildings
9. General panic, considerable damage
10. Destruction of buildings and some bridges
11. Few structures remain standing; railway tracks lifted; water pipelines burst
12. Total damage, large displacements of earth

Cf. earthquake, Richter scale

Mercenary A person recruited to fight in an armed conflict mainly for personal gain, who is neither a national nor a resident of the conflicting countries and is not a member of the armed forces of one of the countries.

Mercy Ships International humanitarian organization providing itinerant medical, surgical and social services through ships that call at ports for aid delivery and health services.
Cf. Peace Boat

Meta-analysis A mathematical statistical approach that synthesises the results of two or more independent primary studies that addressed a given problem or hypothesis in the same way.

Meteorological sounding Determination of the profile of the atmosphere at different altitudes, usually by means of radio or satellite signals.
Cf. ionospheric sounding, remote sounding, WMO, World Weather Watch

Meteorology The science of the atmosphere and of the phenomena that occur in it. Meteorological forecasting can help prevent or mitigate disasters.
Cf. atmosphere

Meteosat The European Geostationary satellite, located above the equator on the prime meridian from where it can observe and transmit images of the meteorological conditions over the whole of Africa, much of Europe and the Atlantic and part of South America. Other operational systems include TIROS-N (USA), METEOR (Russia) and, for hydrology and oceanography, the LANDSAT.
Cf. International Telecommunication Union, meteorology, World Weather Watch, World Meteorological Organization

mHealth An advanced communication technique that harnesses the mobility and timeliness of wireless information and communications technology for health, including instant data transfer between health service providers and patients in various localities – BCMJ. (Not to be confused with eHealth.)

Sn: also m-health, M-health

Cf. eHealth, telemedicine

Microcredit/Microfinance An imaginative and socially conscious financial system that allows poor clients to take out loans at low interest rate that can be used to generate income or to pay for services, such as starting a small business, attending school, skill building, etc. A service used to great advantage in developing countries. Was awarded the 2006 Nobel Peace Prize.

Microzoning Subdividing or mapping of a region into areas or zones where similar hazards or related effects can be expected.

Cf. zonation

Migrant A person who voluntarily moves from one country to another for personal, economic, social, security or political reasons. (Distinguish between emigrant and immigrant.)

Cf. emigrant, immigrant

Migration Movement of people across national regions or international boundaries for the purpose of finding better agricultural or living conditions, or as a result of natural catastrophes or political upheavals.

Cf. emigration, immigration, IOM

Military-industrial complex Powerful economic-industrial-military conglomerate that politically promotes a country's military arms production mainly on the basis of financial gain rather than on defence needs.

Cf. industrial complex

Military conflict A situation characterized by hostilities that bring into opposition two or more organized armies. It constitutes a major man-made disaster.

Cf. Geneva Conventions, International Humanitarian Law, conflict war

Military medicine The art and science of medicine, including in particular, critical care, emergency surgery and traumatology, as applied to mass casualty situations, battlefront conditions, the needs of soldiers and, increasingly, of civilian disaster victims.

Cf. disaster medicine, biological warfare, chemical warfare, nuclear war, triage, GLAWARS Report, WHOPAX Report, CIMIC

Millennium Declaration/UN Cf. Millennium Development Goals

Millennium Development Goals/ MDGs To usher the twenty-first century and improve the developmental process for all peoples, the UN General Assembly adopted the significant 2000 Millennium Declaration and its Millennium Development Goals, to be attained by 2015. The eight specific MDGs represent perceived needs and international commitments to combat poverty and the inequities of underdevelopment. They aim to (1) eradicate extreme poverty and hunger, (2) achieve universal primary education, (3) promote gender equality and empower women, (4) reduce child mortality, (5) improve maternal health, (6) combat HIV/AIDS, malaria and other diseases, (7) ensure environmental sustainability and (8) create partnerships for development. The Goals represent a dynamic process and do not terminate in 2015.

Sn: MDGs, UNMDGs

Millennium Development Project Cf. United Nations Millennium Development Project, Millennium Development Goals

Mines/landmines/antipersonnel mines Treacherous explosive devices used in war, guerrilla strife and terrorism, hidden superficially on roads, passageways and fields and made invisible by covering them with earth. Walking or driving over them triggers a powerful explosion that causes extensive trauma, disability and death. Their existence in millions and the difficulty in defusing them constitute a chronic disaster. The Ottawa Convention prohibits their production and use. The International Campaign to Ban Landmines was awarded the Nobel Peace Prize, 1997.
Cf. Ottawa Convention, ICBL, Cranfield Mine Action

Minorities Community or large group of persons characterized by a sense of separate identity that sets them apart from the larger group in which they live and from which they differ on ethnic, religious or linguistic grounds.
Cf. ethnic group

MIRV In nuclear warfare, acronymic term for Multiple Independently Targeted Re-entry Vehicle, where one missile can carry several warheads directed to different targets.

Missiles/long-range, short-range Cf. antiballistic missiles

Missiles/strategic, non-strategic Cf. antiballistic missiles

Miticide Chemical substance used to destroy mites and other arthropods.
Sn: acaricide
Cf. pesticide

Mitigation A general term for severity reduction, risk diminution, appeasement, alleviation, moderation.
In the context of the wide spectrum of disasters, it describes different approaches to different risks, ranging, inter alia, from general and specific preparedness to citizen education to structural engineering, climatic approaches, planned adaptation, socioeconomic measures, empowerment, etc.
Cf. disaster mitigation, abatement

Mob A tumultuous, disorganized, rowdy assemblage of persons or crowd, with little consideration for law and order. May need to be dispersed by police or other authorities.
Cf. tear gas

Mobile land station Mobile communication station that can move about within a given territory.
Cf. Mobile Satellite Communication System, space station

Mobile Satellite Communication System Communication of necessary detailed information by disaster managers using satellite exchange when other communication facilities have broken down due to the disaster.
Sn: SATCOM
Cf. mobile land station

Molotov cocktail General term for a rather makeshift incendiary device that can be produced easily, cheaply and operated by untrained fighters who cannot afford hand grenades or other weapons. It is roughly produced in a bottle containing a mixture of petrol or alcohol or kerosene, with a soaked wick that on ignition and contact with the targeted object creates a considerable explosion.
Sn: Molotov bomb, petrol bomb, gasoline bomb, fire bottle

Molluscicide Chemical substance used to destroy molluscs (snails).
Cf. pesticide

Monitoring Cf. surveillance, indicators

Monsoon Wind in the general direction of the atmospheric circulation, characterized by a seasonal direction, strongest in the southern and S.E. coasts of Asia and by a marked change of its direction from one season to the other.
Cf. atmosphere, wind

Monsoon climate Type of climate found in regions subject to monsoons, especially around the Indian Ocean, characterized mainly by a dry winter and a wet summer, due to the geographic influences of an unequal warming of the land and of the seas.
Cf. monsoon

Monsoon season In continental regions, the season when the summer monsoon blows. Example: in India.
Cf. summer monsoon

Montreal Protocol International rules and agreement promoted by UNEP beginning in 1980, to diminish chlorofluorocarbons (CFCs) and other ozone-destroying substances in the atmosphere.
Cf. atmospheric pollution

Montreux Document on PMSCs In the field of private military security companies, a Swiss document that sets out the agreed-upon pertinent international legal obligations and good practices for contracting States related to PMSC commercial operations. The five contractants are (a) the "contracting PMSC" business, (b) the personnel of that business, (c) the "contracting State", (d) the "territorial State" on whose territory the personnel operate, (e) the "Home States", where the PMSC business is registered – FDFA.
Cf. private military security company, mercenary

Morbidity
1. The number of sick persons or of diseases in a given period among a given population.
2. The pathological or morbid conditions that characterize a disease, as opposed to mortality that characterizes the killing potentialities of a disease.
Cf. morbidity rate, mortality rate

Morbidity rate
1. For a given disease, the ratio of individuals having that disease to the total number of the population.
2. For a given population, the ratio of all individuals sick from any disease to the total number of the population.
In both cases, the ratio can be expressed as incidence or prevalence.
Cf. death rate, incidence, mortality rate, prevalence

Mortality
1. The number, magnitude or frequency of deaths over a period of time among the total sick and well population of an area.
2. The numerical expression of deaths, usually given as mortality rate.
Cf. morbidity, mortality rate

Mortality rate The ratio of the number of deaths in a given population to the total number of that population.
Sn: death rate
Cf. morbidity rate

Mothballing Cf. sarcophagus

Motivation The reasons, desires and aspirations that determine the behaviour of an individual or a group.

Mountain climate Climate governed by the geographic factor of altitude and characterized by low pressure and by intense solar radiation rich in ultraviolet rays.

Cf. atmospheric pressure

MRSA Short name for methicillin-resistant *Staphylococcus aureus*. Difficult infection to treat.

Mudslide Sn: mud flow
Cf. earth flow, quicksand

Multicultural Youth Council/COJEP French name Conseil de la Jeunesse Pluriculturelle, NGO active in intercultural dialogue issues, human rights, democracy, sound citizenship, struggle against racism and discrimination.

Multilateralism In international and intergovernmental relations, the conduct of negotiations and discussions among multiple (more than two) governments and organizations and not limited to one-to-one (bilateral) discussions or single (unilateral) decisions.
Cf. unilateralism, bilateralism

Multiple organ failure syndrome Very serious condition of an injured patient who, besides severe trauma, e.g. multiple major fractures, or critical illness, e.g. pancreatitis, extensive infection, has involvement of at least two vital organs, e.g. lung and kidney, inducing severe shock and critical state. An early form can follow non-compensated shock, a late form follows multiple infectious insults.
Sn: MOFS

Multisectoral Action or discipline that implies and needs coordination at all levels between and among the various activities involved in managing a situation, e.g. a disaster, such as the health sector, transport, agriculture, housing, public works, water supply, communications, finance, etc.
Sn: intersectoral action, interdisciplinary, multisectoral
Cf. disaster medicine

Mushroom cloud In nuclear war, the characteristic mushroom-shaped cloud composed of hot gases, smoke and other earth particles sucked upwards immediately after the explosion of a nuclear bomb.
Cf. nuclear war, nuclear winter

Mustard gas Dichlorodiethyl sulphide. A lethal and incapacitating, vesicant chemical warfare agent. Notoriously used in World War I with devastating effects.
Cf. chemical weapons, biological weapons, Geneva Protocol

N

Nagasaki (Japan) The second city to suffer an atomic bombardment.
Cf. Hiroshima/Nagasaki

Nansen Passport/Nansen Award Fridtjof Nansen was the first High Commissioner for Refugees. During World War I, with genuine humanitarian spirit and high authority, he helped the victims and the persecuted stateless persons, issuing them with Nansen Passports. A prestigious distinction is now awarded in his memory to men and women who demonstrate exceptional support in favour of the plight of refugees and displaced persons.
Cf. refugee, displaced person, apatride

Napalm Acronymic name for aluminium naphthenate and aluminium palmitate, a chemical fire-producing weapon commonly used as an effective military incendiary bomb.
Cf. Chemical weapons, Geneva Protocol

Narcotraffic Illegal individual or highly organized secret procurement, transport and sale worldwide of narcotics and prohibited drugs, with large sums of money at stake, gang competition, money laundering, mafia activities, powerful antisocial cartels, crime, corruption and government destabilization.

Cf. drug, addiction, mafia, UNODOC

Natural disaster A sudden major upheaval of nature, causing extensive destruction of society, death and suffering among the stricken community and which is not due to man's action. However, (a) some natural disasters can be of slow origin, e.g. drought, and (b) a seemingly natural disaster can be caused or aggravated by man's action, e.g. desertification through excessive land use and deforestation.

A natural hazard does not constitute a natural disaster unless and until it affects man and society. If it does not, it remains a mere natural hazard or a geo-meteorological phenomenon – Gunn.

Cf. disaster, natural hazard, hazard

Natural fire Any fire that is of natural origin that may be caused by lightning, spontaneous combustion or volcanic eruption.

Natural hazard The probability of occurrence, within a specific period of time in a given area, of a potentially damaging phenomenon of nature – UN.

It remains a hazard, and not a disaster, until it affects man and society.

Cf. natural disaster, hazard

Natural phenomenon Cf. natural disaster (Part II), natural hazard

Natural resources The aggregate of mineral and biotic elements of the earth, as well as the various forms of energy occurring in the natural state (solar energy) or environmental forces independent of man (winds, tides), that is considered as being of potential value to man. Natural resources can be:

– Renewable, by reproduction (living organisms) or by biogeochemical cycles (water, nitrogen)
– Non-renewable (petrol)
– Permanent (solar energy)

Natural resources management Administration of the natural resources in a manner that promotes judicious utilization, conservation and renewal, with minimum waste, pollution or depletion, for the improvement of disaster management.

Cf. natural resources

Near-field In a nuclear incident, the immediate zone, extending from some 5–20 km, around the damaged plant that is considered most dangerous and is cordoned off until further notice. The relatively less dangerous area beyond is called "far-field".

Cf. far-field, nuclear accident, ground zero, zone zero

Needs The sum of the biological, social, psychological and physical elements necessary, at a given time, for the well-being, existence and even survival of the individual or society.

Cf. well-being, sustainable development

Neglected tropical diseases A group of communicable diseases that thrive in unsanitary, impoverished settings and further contribute to sickness, poverty and underdevelopment. WHO lists 17 such neglected diseases: dengue, rabies, trachoma, buruli ulcer, endemic treponematoses, leprosy, Chagas disease, sleeping sickness, leishmaniasis, cysticercosis, dracunculiasis, echinococcosis, food-borne trematodes, lymphatic filariasis, onchocerciasis, schistosomiasis, soil transmitted helminthiases.

Sn: orphan diseases

Cf. these diseases separately. Millennium Development Goals, poverty

Nematocide Medicament used to kill nematodes – intestinal and tissue worms, like the pinworm, whipworm, hookworm, ascarids, toxocara, filariae, onchocerca.

Cf. parasite, pesticide

Neocolonialism A deprecatory term referring to the dominant involvement of developed countries in the affairs of developing (mainly African and particularly ex-colonial) countries through direct or indirect paternalistic, economic, neo-imperialistic, political and cultural means.

Cf. colonialism

Nephanalysis System of meteorological information gathering based on the study of the clouds, usually seen from above.

Cf. meteorology

Nepotism Undeserved favours and patronage given to relatives and close friends in return for advantages, loyalty and security.

Nerve gas/Nerve agent Dangerous and potentially lethal organophosphorus compounds that inhibit tissue cholinesterase. Used in chemical warfare to incapacitate the enemy by interfering with the nerve impulses of the victim. The two main families are the G and V agents. Weapons of mass destruction.

Sn: Agent G, Agent V

Cf. chemical weapons, sarin, CBW, Geneva Protocol

Nine/Eleven (9/11) Sn: September 11, 2001 (the New York disaster)

Niño Cf. El Niño

Nippon Foundation Established in 1962 by Ryoichi Sasakawa, important Japanese foundation with extensive international humanitarian action in health, sciences, youth education and social studies. Has established a prize for disaster work and is WHO goodwill ambassador for leprosy.

Nobel Prize The most distinguished prize, established by the Swedish industrialist Alfred Nobel (1833–1896), awarded annually to persons who have made the greatest contribution to mankind in specific fields of medicine, science, economics, literature and humanitarian work.

The first Nobel Prize for Peace (Pro Pace et Fraternitate Gentium) was given in 1901 to Henry Dunant, founder of the International Committee of the Red Cross, and in the same year, the first Nobel Prize for Medicine or Physiology was awarded to Wilhelm Röntgen for his work on X-rays. The Peace Prize has also been awarded to the United Nations and its Secretary-General Kofi Annan in recognition of humanitarian services in favour of world peace and to Pugwash and its President Joseph Rotblat for their efforts against nuclear war.

Cf. Red Cross, Pugwash

Nomad The traditional way of life in certain rural people who do not live continually in the same area but move cyclically or periodically, usually in search of grazing or hunting grounds and watering places, or financial opportunities, and who are well adapted to their changing environment.

There are also ethnically nomad groups, such as Romanies, Sintis, Gypsies, Tsiganes.

Cf. migration, population mobility, Tsiganes, Roma, gypsies

Non-governmental organization (NGO) A private, civil society, international, not governmental organization (as distinct from an intergovernmental or governmental organization), constituted as a single association or as a federation of various national organizations, without governmental or state ties. The most important NGOs are given consultative status with the United Nations or its specialized agencies and are active in disasters, civil society services and humanitarian aid. Examples: MSF, International Association for Humanitarian Medicine, Medicus Mundi, AI.
Cf. civil society, voluntary agency, non-state health actors

Non-international armed conflict Cf. civil war

Non-refoulement Cf. principle of non-refoulement

Non-state health actors Long time the prerogative of Ministries of Health and major intergovernmental organizations, health is becoming increasingly the subject of interest and intervention at higher non-governmental, non-state levels. Quite distinct from the very useful traditional inputs of a multitude of NGOs, powerful, wealthy, knowledgeable and well-informed non-state institutions, such as the Bill and Melinda Gates Foundation, the Wellcome Trust, the Bill Clinton Foundation and others, are becoming indispensable health actors.

Non-structural elements In a building, those parts of the construction (e.g. partitions, ceilings) that are not components of the load-bearing system. Strict construction codes regulate the necessary requirements for structural elements, e.g. for earthquake resistance.

Non-tropical cyclone Sn: depression

Non-violence A personal belief and posture that war is a bad and wrong thing and that progress and freedom can be achieved and maintained without resorting to violent action, whether at the personal or national level. Mahatma Gandhi and Nelson Mandela have proven this. Also written non violence.
Cf. war, violence

North Atlantic Treaty Organization/ NATO Commonly referred to as NATO, an alliance established in accordance with the United Nations Charter, to ensure security through defensive, political, military and scientific ties among its members.
Cf. European Union, United Nations, OSCE

North–South A theoretical, artificial division of the globe into North, representing the developed, more affluent, technologically advanced, financially rich, healthy, educated and stable countries, and South, with developing, poor, indebted, technologically retarded countries where mortality is high, health levels low and education deficient. The gap between north and south is disastrous.
Cf. development

Nosocomial infection An infection or disease acquired during a stay in hospital.
Cf. iatrogenic disease

Note verbale A diplomatic note, which is in fact not verbal but written, exchanged between diplomatic missions and intergovernmental organizations. Most commonly, it is used by the diplomatic representative

resident in a country with the Minister of Foreign Affairs of the host country. It is customarily written in the third person.
Cf. protocol

Notifiable disease A disease that by law or decree must be reported to a government health authority.

Nuclear accident Unintentional, accidental release of radiation or radioactive material in or around a civil nuclear facility, exceeding the internationally set safety levels.
A less severe of such event is referred to as a nuclear incident.
Cf. radiation injury, radiation protection, radioactive decontamination, Chernobyl

Nuclear activity The number of spontaneous nuclear disintegrations within a radionuclide at any given time. The old unit of activity, the curie (Ci) has been replaced by the becquerel (Bq).
Cf. becquerel

Nuclear cloud Sn: radioactive cloud
Cf. fallout

Nuclear energy Energy liberated in nuclear reactions, especially in fission or fusion reactions.

Nuclear fallout Sn: radioactive fallout
Cf. fallout

Nuclear famine The climatic consequences of nuclear war would create abrupt global cooling, with alteration of precipitation patterns, radioactive contamination and major crop failures, leading to global famine, starvation, exposure to cold weather, major epidemics and social violence.
Cf. nuclear war, nuclear winter, GLAWARS

Nuclear fuel Material containing fissile nuclides which when placed in a reactor enables a self-sustaining nuclear chain reaction to be achieved.
Cf. fissile uranium

Nuclear hazard(s) Radioactive material is potentially hazardous, both as a military nuclear weapon (atomic war, e.g. Hiroshima) and in civilian activities (e.g. Chernobyl). A peacetime nuclear plant has the following potentials for disaster: a meltdown and disintegration, releasing massive amounts of radioactivity (Chernobyl); effluent leaks from plant weaknesses; radioactive waste accumulation, as no safe disposal exists; plutonium production, which is a hazard and raw material for atomic bomb production; radioactive release into the atmosphere and environment, with absorption into food, inhalation and ingestion.
Cf. Chernobyl, Fukushima, Three Mile Island, fallout, plutonium, nuclear reprocessing

Nuclear incident Cf. nuclear accident

Nuclear meltdown Cf. meltdown, nuclear accident

Nuclear nomads hazard A nondescript mass of nuclear personnel who, quite distinct from the highly specialized established scientists, represent a non-organized body of less trained but needed, mobile seasonal employees such as electricians, plumbers, solderers, underwater workers, etc., who move uncontrolled from one nuclear facility to another as jobs open up, in the meantime constituting a potential nuclear hazard.

Nuclear Non-Proliferation Treaty/ NPT Treaty formulated in 1970 to prevent the further spread of nuclear weapons, to foster peaceful nuclear cooperation under safeguards, to encourage ending the nuclear arms race, non-nuclear states not to produce arms and to aspire to complete nuclear disarmament.

Cf. SALT, START

Nuclear power station Cf. reactor

Nuclear radiation effects

1. Genetic: Change of hereditary character caused by ionizing radiation.
2. Somatic: Effects of radiation that appear in the lifetime of an exposed subject.

Cf. radioactive contamination

Nuclear reaction Disintegration and change in the nucleus of an atom induced by bombarding it with a radioactive particle, with liberation of energy.

Cf. nuclear activity

Nuclear reactor An industrial system for generating heat and electricity from nuclear power by controlled fission of uranium-235 (fission reaction) or by the fusion of light atoms (fusion reaction).

Generally intended for peaceful, civilian uses of nuclear energy, but accidents, e.g. Chernobyl, Fukushima, can be a disaster with immediate and long-lasting effects.

Sn: nuclear power plant, atomic reactor, atomic power plant

CF. Chernobyl, Fukushima, Three Mile Island, International Atomic Energy Agency, nuclear accident

Nuclear reactor dismantling/decommissioning Dismantling means planned total structural demolition and stoppage of a facility. Decommissioning is discontinuing the services of a facility. For nuclear reactors, either action is risky, dangerous and difficult. Following the Fukushima disaster of 2011, several countries have decided to discontinue

the use of nuclear power and are proceeding to staged decommissioning and dismantling (deconstruction) of their reactors. At every stage, there are risks, and even after total clearance, radioactivity persists. Karlsruhe Institute of Technology is specialized in dismantling. The French Superphenix was stopped in 1997 and full deconstruction will not be completed before 2028.

Cf. Fukushima, Fukushima effect, nuclear accident, reactor

Nuclear reprocessing Reprocessing is the chemical separation of plutonium and unburnt uranium – and to a lesser extent caesium and other radioactive isotopes – from the spent fuel rods of a nuclear reactor. The process creates large amounts of radioactive waste in three forms: (a) gaseous, with radioactivity in the environment, (b) solids in earth dumps and (c) marine discharges, all highly dangerous for generations to come.

Cf. nuclear hazards, uranium, Sellafield, Basel Convention, La Hague, International Atomic Energy Agency.

Nuclear safety All decisions and measures taken to protect workers, people and property from the harmful effects of radiation contamination, exposure to ionizing radiation and nuclear criticality.

Cf. radioactive decontamination, International Atomic Energy Agency, sustainable elimination

Nuclear war War in which nuclear weapons – as opposed to conventional explosive devices – are used. Like conventional bombs, nuclear weapons produce extensive blast and fire damage, but to an infinitely higher degree. Furthermore, the immediate power of a nuclear explosion is increased by the following factors: intense radiation at the time of the explosion, lasting for about one minute; intense heat and light from the fireball, lasting a few seconds; local radioactive fallout and a strong electromagnetic radiation. Later effects add to the devastation. The nuclear bomb used on Nagasaki was 2,200 times more powerful than the largest conventional weapon used in World War II.

Sn: atomic war

Cf. atomic bomb, fission bomb, fusion bomb, hydrogen bomb, NPT, START, electromagnetic pulse, nuclear winter, nuclear weapon, zero option

Nuclear waste Cf. waste, nuclear reprocessing, Sellafield, La Hague

Nuclear weapon Generic term for any weapon based on nuclear explosion. The atom bomb is a nuclear weapon that derives its energy from fission of heavy elements, mainly uranium or plutonium; the hydrogen bomb derives its energy mainly from fusion.

Cf. atomic bomb, hydrogen bomb, weapons of mass destruction

Nuclear winter A term that describes the very damaging climatic and environmental situation likely to result from reduced sunlight and lowered temperatures following nuclear war.

Cf. firestorm, mushroom cloud, nuclear war, nuclear famine, GLAWARS

Nuée ardente Sn: glowing cloud

Nuremberg Charter/Law – International crimes In 1945, the Charter identified three classes of international crimes: crimes against peace, war crimes, crimes against humanity. Established the legal basis of international crimes committed by individuals or groups.

Cf. Nuremberg Code/medical

Nuremberg Code Following the 1947 trials of the Nazi war criminals, along with other international ethical prescriptions, a code of ethical conduct in medicine was also established, dealing in particular with research involving humans. Ten standards are laid down to which physicians must conform. The Code stipulates that "the voluntary consent of the subject is absolutely essential". This has now extended beyond research and is valid for all interventions in humans.

Cf. Helsinki Declaration, informed consent, consent

Nutrient Any and all of the organic compounds and mineral salts contained in foods and water which are utilized in the normal metabolism of the body and play a specific role in nutrition and growth.

All nutrients consist of a combination of (a) macronutrients that produce energy: proteins, fats, carbohydrates and (b) micronutrients: vitamins and minerals essential to life.

In poorer developing countries, carbohydrates are the main source of energy (80%) and fats (8–10%). Micronutrient deficiency concerns some two billion people – WFP.

Cf. food, nutrition

Nutrition

1. The function of assimilation and metabolism whereby living organisms utilize food for maintenance of life.

2. In public health, the discipline that deals with the interactions of food, health, disease and the improvement of health standards through

prevention and treatment of nutritional diseases.

Cf. deficiency disease, food health

Nutrition evaluation Evaluation of the nutritional state of persons and of the community and estimation of food needs according to criteria based on nutritional indicators.

Cf. nutrition indicators

Nutrition indicators Calculations that permit to evaluate in quantified terms the nutritional changes that have occurred in a given population. Two kinds of indicators can be distinguished: food and nutrition indicators and indicators of the state of nutrition.

Cf. food and nutrition indicators, nutrition, nutritional state indicators, evaluation

Nutritional cachexia Sn: nutritional marasmus

Nutritional deficiency Absence or insufficiency, in the food or in the organism, of elements indispensable for nutrition.

Cf. nutrition, malnutrition, vitamin deficiency

Nutritional marasmus Severe form of protein-calorie malnutrition occurring mainly in infants, characterized by wasting, retardation of growth and cachexia. Other factors such as infection and infestation can play a role in its aetiology and aggravation.

Sn: athrepsy, nutritional cachexia.

Cf. kwashiorkor, marasmus, protein-calorie malnutrition

Nutritional requirements The amount of energy and nutrients normally calculated on averages and expressed on a daily basis, which cover the needs of healthy individuals or groups for growth and for the normal function of the body.

Cf. needs

Nutritional state evaluation Measurement and assessment, according to specific indices and criteria, of the nutritional condition of a given population, e.g. children, the elderly, new immigrants, expectant mothers, etc. in normal times, in emergencies or after a disaster, with the view to correcting any deficiencies.

Cf. nutritional state indicators, nutrition indicators

Nutritional state indicators Physical, functional and biochemical measurements used to describe with precision the nutritional state of persons or a population group and to quantify the changes that have occurred.

Cf. food and nutrition indicators, nutritional indicators

O

Obesity Overweight. Abnormal or excessive accumulation of fat that presents a health risk. One measure is the body mass index (BMI). A person with a BMI equal to or more than 30 is obese, BMI equal to or more than 25 is overweight and above 40 is pathological. All are risk factors. Obesity is a danger not only in affluent circles but also in disaster situations and refugee camps due to the wrong nutrition.

Cf. malnutrition, body mass index

Objective The end result that a programme or an aim seeks to achieve. For example, the objective of community education for disaster preparedness can be defined as ensuring that people in risk areas will want to be less vulnerable, know how to act in case of disaster, do what they can individually and collectively at the time of emergency and do the necessary before the emergency so that they can be prepared for it.

Cf. goal, plan, target, MDGs

Obninsk The Hospital at Obninsk, near Moscow, that continues to receive and treat great numbers of direct, indirect and distant victims of radiation since 1986 from the Chernobyl nuclear disaster.
Cf. Chernobyl, radiation injury, thyroid

Ocean wave A wave system generated by winds at some distance from the coast over a wide area, with little change in its characteristics.
Cf. seismic sea wave, storm wave, swell, tsunami

Oceanic Describes the marine area beyond the coast, generally situated away from the continental margin.

Oceanic ridge Submarine elevation along several thousand kilometres, with deep reliefs resulting from the rising of the crust.
Cf. ridge, submarine ridge

Oceanology The exploration and scientific study of the oceans and the seas (oceanography) and the techniques of protection and management of marine sources.

Office for the Coordination of Humanitarian Affairs (OCHA) Special focal point in the UN Department of Humanitarian Affairs (DHA) to mobilize, direct, and coordinate the emergency humanitarian activities of the various UN agencies and other organizations, particularly in response to disasters. Previously UNDRO.
Cf. United Nations, ISDR

Office of the High Commissioner for Human Rights (OHCHR) The United Nations central point for all human rights questions. Leads and stimulates human rights issues, responds to serious violations of human rights, investigates reports on their breaches, promotes human rights, strengthens national action in their favour and ensures that UN decisions on human rights are implemented and the articles of the Universal Declaration of Human Rights respected.
Cf. human rights, Universal Declaration of Human Rights, United Nations, IAHM

Office of the UN Disaster Relief Co-ordinator (UNDRO) Superseded by United Nations Office for the Coordination of Humanitarian Affairs (OCHA).
Cf. Office for the Coordination of Humanitarian Affairs

Office of Special Relief Operations/OSRO The emergency assistance department of the UN Food and Agriculture Organization.
Cf. humanitarian assistance, food aid

Office of US Foreign Disaster Assistance (OFDA) Within the US Agency for International Development, OFDA is responsible for providing non-food, humanitarian assistance in international crises and disasters. It is part of the Bureau for Humanitarian Affairs (BHR), with four divisions: disaster response; prevention; mitigation, preparedness and planning; operational support; programme support.
Cf. humanitarian assistance, international assistance, USAID

Offshore wind Wind that engenders the surface movement of the water towards the open sea (as opposed to onshore wind).
Cf. onshore wind, wind

Oil boom Sn: floating barrier
Cf. oil slick, oil spill, black tide

Oil pollution Pollution of the oceans, lakes and rivers by discharge of hydrocarbon products, mostly petroleum, crude oil, during offshore drilling, transportation or storage, from platforms, tanks, tankers or pipelines. The most devastating pollution due to oil spill from failure of a platform occurred in April 2010 off Louisiana, USA.

Cf. black tide, oil slick, floating barrier, technological disaster

Oil slick Oil, discharged naturally, by accident or intentionally, floating on the water and carried by wind, currents and tides. A more serious amount of oil slick, with tar balls and oil deposits on tidelands, is called black tide. Disastrous examples are the Exxon-Valdes tanker break-up in Alaska, the British Petroleum spill in the Louisiana Gulf region.

Sn: black tide

Cf. oil pollution, tar balls, floating barrier

Oil spill Cf. oil pollution, oil slick

Onchocerciasis A filarial infection caused by *Onchocerca volvulus* and spread by the *Simulid* blackfly. It is characterized by nodules in the skin and subcutaneous tissues, but its most serious complication is blindness, with subsequent socio-economic disaster. Common in sub-Saharan Africa and South America, along river basins. WHO has a long-term anti-onchocerciasis programme and the availability of ivermectin for this neglected tropical disease.

Sn: river blindness

Cf. filariasis, parasitic diseases, neglected tropical diseases

Onshore wind Wind that engenders the surface movement of the sea towards the coast (as opposed to offshore wind).

Cf. offshore wind

Open sea Sn: high seas

Optional Protocol Against Torture/ OPCAT More correctly, Optional Protocol to the UN Convention Against Torture, adopted in 2002 by the UN General Assembly, with the aim of preventing torture and other forms of ill-treatment by a system of regular inspections.

Cf. torture, places of torture detention

Oral rehydration Providing a dehydrated person, e.g. suffering from diarrhoea, with the necessary fluids and electrolytes by mouth. In severe cases, rehydration may be necessary by the intravenous route.

Cf. diarrhoea, oral rehydration salts, dehydration

Oral rehydration salts (ORS) Convenient and effective means of providing fluids and electrolytes to a dehydrated person. The proven WHO/UNICEF formula of ORS comes in 27,5 g sachets, as follows:

Sodium chloride (common salt) 3.5 g

Glucose 20.0 g

Sodium bicarbonate 2.5 g

Potassium chloride 1.5 g

To be diluted in 1 l of clean drinking water.

Sn: ORS

Cf. diarrhoea, oral rehydration, dehydration

Orderly departure

1. Organized displacement or departure of refugees or victims of a disaster.
2. The UNHCR programme for orderly departure is based on a memorandum of understanding concluded by the HCR and the government concerned, establishing the procedures for the departure of the refugee who possesses an exit visa from the country and a resettlement guarantee from the host country.

Cf. refugee

Organization of activities In refugee or displaced communities, the planning and organization of time for productive and educational purposes, besides recuperation and recreational (leisure) activities.
Cf. organization of leisure

Organization of leisure Planning and implementation of recreational activities within a social and environmental programme.
Cf. organization of activities

Organized crime Cf. Palermo Convention Against Organized Crime

Oroya fever Sn: bartonellosis

Orphan diseases/Orphan drugs Diseases that are rare and of low prevalence, attracting little attention and neglected by the scientific and medical communities, by the authorities and by the pharmaceutical industry. There are currently an estimated 6,000 such orphan or rare diseases. Because of their rarity and little financial profitability, the health industry also remains disinterested, thus resulting in orphan drugs.
Somewhat akin to but not to be confused with forgotten diseases.
Cf. neglected tropical diseases

Oslo Treaty Treaty signed in 2008 prohibiting cluster bombs.
Cf. cluster bomb, Ottawa Treaty

Ottawa Charter Significant international declaration (1986) on health promotion.

Ottawa Treaty International Convention to Ban Landmines that entered into force on 1 March 1999, making it illegal to produce, sell, stockpile or use landmines/antipersonnel mines and requiring all states to clear mines, destroy stocks and support victims. Such mines cause extensive damage indiscriminately, trauma and deaths, and their persisting numbers in millions constitute a chronic disaster. The Nobel Peace Prize was awarded to ICBL in recognition of the struggle against landmines.
Cf. mines, Oslo Treaty

Outcome The resultant of planned projects and interventions in relation to pre-established actions, expected goals and objectives.

Outer Space Treaty International Treaty signed in 1987, prohibiting the placing of any weapons of mass destruction in outer space.
Cf. star wars, arsenalization of space, strategic defence initiative

Outrage, Time for Cf. Indignez Vous!

Overflow Flooding or the spilling phase of a swell during which the abundant waters are liable to reshape the surface of the flooded area by furrowing, cutting out hollows or depositing alluvium.
Cf. alluvium, flood, swell

Overnutrition Sn: hypernutrition
Cf. malnutrition

Overpressure Transient increase, beyond the normal atmospheric pressure, in the blast wave that follows a nuclear explosion.

Overspill Permanent change in the course of a stream or river which, due to spilling over, changes its bed and follows another course.
Sn: spill

Ovicide Medicament or chemical substance intended to kill the ova or eggs of parasites.
Cf. pesticide

Oxfam The Oxford Committee for Famine Relief. Started in 1942, it has grown far beyond famine assistance and is at present one of the most important, efficient, ethical international humanitarian NGOs and providers of assistance in any major disaster worldwide.

Oxyology A new term (not much used) for emergency medicine involving rapid response, first aid, triage, transport, resuscitation and urgent care.

Sn: Emergency Medical Services, disastrology

Cf. CPR, disaster medicine, first aid, triage

Ozone An unstable molecular form of oxygen that consists of three atoms (O_3). Present in the lower layers of the stratosphere, about 20–50 km above the earth's surface, it protects the earth from excessive solar radiation. Certain chemical pollutants can cause depletion of the layer, with resulting global environmental damage.

Sn: ozonosphere Cf. ozone depletion, chlorofluorocarbons

Ozone depletion The stratospheric ozone layer that protects the earth from excessive ultraviolet radiations can be depleted by certain pollutants. Gases used in spray cans (chlorofluorocarbons, chlorofluoromethanes) or oxides of nitrogen released by cars and flying aircraft can damage or create "holes" in the ozone layer, allowing excess amounts of ultraviolet radiation to reach the earth, with global climatic and environmental consequences and damage to health. A combined technological and natural disaster.

Sn: ozone hole

Cf. chlorofluorocarbons, glasshouse effect, ozone, global warming, Kyoto protocol, World Meteorological Organization, United Nations Environment Programme, climate change

P

Pacifism A doctrine and personal view that war is wrong, that international disputes can be solved peacefully and that military and war instruments are unnecessary and should be abolished. Not to be confused with non-violence.

Cf. war, non-violence, conscientious objector

Pack ice Sn: ice pack

Palermo Convention against Organized Crime International agreement signed in Palermo, Italy, 2000, under the aegis of the United Nations, banning the mafia, transnational racketeering, money laundering, trafficking in humans, drug cartels and other illicit activities constituting organized crime.

Cf. mafia, disappearances, man-conceived disaster, narcotraffic

Palliative treatment Treatment and comforting help given to reduce pain, alleviate immobility or relieve other symptoms of a disease, but not to cure the disease.

Cf. hospice

Palmer drought index A mathematical formula indicating drought conditions.

Cf. aridity, famine, Sahel

Pandemic The presence of a disease in important proportions at the same time throughout the world. Example: AIDS.

Cf. endemicity, epidemic

Panic Acute and overwhelming sense of fear and dread, usually of sudden onset and most often self-limiting and of short duration, from a few seconds to hours, accompanying restlessness resulting in an urge to escape. A frequent but not lasting phenomenon, following disasters and major emergencies.

Paragrapher Vessel of less than 500 tons usually used for coastal or inshore navigation that can be utilized in emergencies with a small crew, life-saving equipment and light radio facilities.

Parasitic diseases Infections, infestation and other disease states caused by parasites of animal origin. Some examples common in disaster situations are amoebiasis, intestinal worms, schistosomiasis, malaria, trypanosomiasis, scabies, pediculosis.

Paris Declaration The Paris Declaration on Aid Effectiveness, signed in 2005, seeks to enable aid-recipient countries rather than donors "to execute their own national plans according to their own national priorities ... on long term" and be mutually accountable.
Cf. Accra Agenda

Participation The philosophy and action of taking part in a decision-making process, being responsible for one's contribution and sharing the burden.

Pathogen(ic) Bacterium, virus, prion, parasite, fungus or other microorganisms that can cause disease.

Pathogenicity
1. Capacity to cause disease.
2. Which carries a pathogen.
Cf. pathogen

Pathology
1. The medical science that studies disease.
2. By extension, it is also commonly but erroneously used to mean disease or the characteristics of a disease.

Patient A sick person who needs, is receiving or will receive medical care, treatment or surgical attention.

Peace Boat A Japan-based but international NGO that works to promote peace, human rights and environmental development by making calls at various ports where advocacy and teaching are promoted.
Cf. Mercy Ship

Peace Corps A US governmental humanitarian agency that conducts international assignments and carries out voluntary services in developing countries.

Pediculosis Infestation by lice. The condition is facilitated by overcrowding and poor sanitary conditions. Lice may cause or transmit infection.
Cf. infestation, louse infestation

Pellagra Disease due to deficiency of vitamin PP or niacin, usually endemic in areas where maize or millet forms the major part of the diet. It is characterized by skin rash, diarrhoea and mental retardation.
Sn: hypovitaminosis PP
Cf. hypovitaminosis, vitamin deficiency

People's Health Movement A civil society organization that promotes health through searching for alternative world solutions, a vision of equity, human rights and peoples' empowerment. Publishes the "Global Health Watch".

Perinatal mortality The death of the foetus after a gestation of 22 weeks.

Permafrost A surface layer of frosted soil and rock with a continuous temperature below 0 °C for several years.

Persona non grata Diplomatic expression indicating that a person representing his State or organization in a host country is no more desirable or welcome and must leave.

Pertussis Sn: whooping cough
Cf. Expanded Programme on Immunization

Pest control Technique aimed at inhibiting the growth and stopping the spread of parasites and other pests.

Pesticide Chemical compound used for killing organisms that are dangerous, undesirable or a nuisance to man, animals or plants. They are named according to their action, such as fungicide, herbicide, insecticide, molluscicide, nematocide, ovicide, rodenticide, virucide. (The suffix -cide means which kills.)

Pharaonic circumcision Sn: infibulation, female genital mutilation

Phases of disaster A disaster can be phased in chronological order, e.g. pre-event status, preparedness, warning, threat, impact, rescue, reconstruction, rehabilitation.
Recently, a psychological behavioural phasing has been suggested in the US: heroic phase, honeymoon phase, disillusionment phase, reconstruction phase – DHHS.

Philanthrocapitalism A new journalistic term for a business-like approach to charity, as extremely rich philanthropic capitalists, e.g. Bill Gates, promote worthy causes, such as health, with huge donations – after *Time*.
Cf. Bill and Melinda Gates Foundation, philanthropy

Philanthropic foundations Organizations that derive their capital from large bequests and/or donations and disburse funds to causes that fit their aims – Last.
Examples of health benefactors: Rockefeller Foundation, Ford Foundation, Gulbenkian Foundation, Carnegie Corporation, the Wellcome Trust, Bill and Melinda Gates Foundation.

Philanthropy Love and practical benevolence towards humanity, desire to help mankind and share one's advantages with fellow beings.

Phosgene A lethal, lung irritant agent used as chemical weapon.
Cf. chemical warfare, Geneva Protocol, CBW

Pinta A serious treponema infection endemic to hot and humid forest regions.
Cf. yaws

Piracy Violent action, for private ends, committed on the high seas outside the jurisdiction of a state. It is an offence under international law.
Cf. high seas, hacking
Piracy of electronic information is hacking.

Places of torture detention Places of detention where torture may be practised and that can be visited for inspection according to the UN Convention Against Torture should include police stations, security force stations, all pretrial centres, remand prisons, prisons for sentenced persons, centres for juveniles, immigration centres, transit zones at ports, centres for detained asylum seekers, psychiatric institutions and places of administrative detention – OPCAT.
Cf. torture, Optional Protocol on Torture

Plague A highly dangerous contagious disease, often fatal if untreated, caused by the *bacillus pestis*, transmitted by infected rats and rodents, through flea bites or at times by airborne spread (pneumonic plague). Overcrowding, unsanitary conditions and large food stores encourage rat proliferation, the vector.

Sn: black death, bubonic plague, pestis

Plan A pre-established course of action which, when implemented, is expected to lead to the attainment of the expected ends and objectives. An orderly set of decisions on the ways and means to achieving the impact and objectives sought.

Cf. goal, objective, target, outcome

Plate tectonics Tectonics is the branch of geological science that deals with regional structural and deformational aspects of the earth's crust. Plate tectonics refers to the concept that the crust consists of several large geological rigid plates whose borders represent fault zones along which slipping movements, deformity and earthquake activity occur.

Cf. earthquake, fault, transform fault, tsunami

Pledging conference Any conference called specifically to present a programme and obtain pledges of financial support for its realization. The phrase is, however, most commonly used for the Ad Hoc Committee of the General Assembly for the announcement of voluntary contributions to the programme of the United Nations High Commissioner for Refugees.

Sn: donors' meeting

Cf. donor, request for disaster assistance

Plutocracy The ruling class of the wealthy, unsocial government dictated by riches and the influence of money.

Cf. autocracy, democracy, kleptocracy

Plutonium Plutonium 239 is an artificially created (1941) fissile material, the product of bombarding uranium with neutrons. It is used in nuclear bombs and nuclear power; the Nagasaki atomic bomb was of the plutonium type. Being relatively inexpensive to produce, it has contributed to the proliferation of nuclear weapons since 1945.

Cf. uranium, caesium, atom bomb, Sellafield, SALT

Pluviometry Sn: rainfall amount

Pogrom Russian word for organized persecution and massacre, especially of the opponents of the regime.

Cf. concentration camp, Auschwitz, ethnic cleansing

Polder A low-lying humid region, protected artificially against the surrounding waters by structures that can also be used for regulating the water levels. Example: Holland.

Policy A set of objectives, course of action or a road map, reflecting certain principles considered to be useful, helpful and advantageous in guiding the authorities and associated persons or organization to achieve the agreed desired goals.

Poliomyelitis An acute viral contagious infection which begins with fever, headache, stiff neck and back, but predominantly settles in the central nervous system, especially the spinal cord, causing paralysis. Epidemic outbreaks are to be feared in unsanitary and disaster conditions. Vaccination prevents the disease and is included in the WHO thrust and Expanded Programme on Immunization.

Sn: infantile paralysis, polio

Pollution Degradation of one or more elements or aspects in the environment by noxious industrial, chemical or biological wastes, from debris of man-made products and from mismanagement of natural and environmental resources.

Cf. air pollution, atmospheric pollution, man-made disaster, oil pollution.

Pontifical Council of the Pastoral Staff for Health Professionals Pontificio Consiglio della Pastorale per gli Operatori Sanitari.

The Vatican's equivalent of Ministry of Health. Includes Cor Unum, for Coordination of Roman Catholic Relief Agencies.

Population The aggregate of individuals belonging to several biological species of the same systematic group that occupies a given territory. Examples: avian population, rodent population.

Population at risk A defined group of people or community threatened by a potential hazard, e.g. a nearby volcano, a polder or a nuclear station, whose lives, livelihood and property may be at risk at any time.

Population concentration Sn: demographic concentration

Population density The number of persons per a given area of land, such as square kilometre. It expresses the extent and distribution of the population of a region.

Cf. demography

Population dynamics Study, in a given space and time, of the mechanisms and changes of population structures and the factors that determine those changes.

Cd. demography

Population mobility The characteristic of a defined group of people likely to change its place of residence, expressed by the frequency of such displacements.

Cf. migration, nomad, Roma

Population service International/PSI A non-profit NGO which, together with Malaria No More, is the world's major distributor of anti-malarial mosquito nets and aims at ending malaria in Africa by 2015.

Portable nuclear arm Stolen or clandestine nuclear device secretly carried (nuclear bag) for illegal arms sales, sabotage or terrorist attacks.

Sn: bag bomb

Cf. atom bomb, terrorism

Post-traumatic stress disorder/syndrome Delayed or protracted reaction to an exceptionally strong stressful event of catastrophic dimension which can cause pervasive distress in almost any person, but more marked in some, following a natural or man-made disaster, combat, violent death, torture, rape, terrorism, etc. The onset may follow the trauma within a few weeks or at most six months. Typical symptoms include "reliving" or "flashbacks" of the event, "numbness" and detachment and fearful reminiscences.

Sn: also called post-traumatic stress syndrome, PTSS, PTSD

Cf. panic, stupor, stress, shock

Potable water Sn: drinking water

Potential epidemic Sn: threatened epidemic

Poverty A human condition characterized by sustained or chronic deprivation of the resources, capabilities, choices, security and power necessary for the enjoyment of an adequate standard of living and other civil, cultural, economic, political and social rights – UN.

Income calculated at less than $2 a day per person. The UN Millennium Development Goals have made it a priority to diminish poverty and its multidimensional consequences worldwide.

Cf. Millennium Development Goals, low-income country, LDC, pro-poor health approach

Poverty reduction strategy Investigations and resulting strategy papers prepared by countries through a participatory process that brings together national stakeholders, external development partners, the World Bank, the International Monetary Fund and other experts with the view to advising and guiding on poverty and poverty reduction issues. These useful strategy papers (PRSPs) are updated every 3 years.

Cf. poverty, low-income country, pro-poor health, MDGs

Precipitation All or any form of water, in liquid or solid state, whether rain, snow, drizzle, sleet, hail, that falls from the atmosphere onto the earth's surface.

Cf. fall

Precursor, seismic Sn: foreshock

Cf. aftershock, earthquake

Precursors, volcanic Rumbling and phenomena indicating a probable volcanic eruption.

Prediction A statement giving the expected time, place and magnitude of a future disruptive event, such as a volcanic eruption or earthquake. (Forecasting is used for the weather.)

Cf. precursor

Prehospital medicine The system and provision of basic emergency treatment to persons who have suffered a sudden illness or injury outside the availability of a hospital or organized medical services and rendered by competent persons with the intention of preventing disability or death and ensuring safe transfer to a hospital or other appropriate facility.

Sn: emergency medical services, EMS

Preparedness Cf. disaster preparedness

Press freedom Cf. freedom of the press, Windhoek Declaration

Prevalence The number of illnesses, accidents or sick persons in a given population and time, without distinction between new and old cases. Cf. incidence

Prevention Medicine: Approaches and activities aimed at reducing the likelihood that a disease will affect the individual, interrupting or slowing the progress of the disease and strengthening health.

Law and society: Laws, governance and activities aimed at reducing the likelihood of lawlessness and disorder in a community and promoting a state of safe, equitable and harmonious living.

Prevention (of disaster) Cf. disaster prevention

Primary health care/PHC Essential health care made universally accessible to individuals and families in the community by means acceptable to them, through their full participation and at a cost that the community and country can afford and sustain. It forms an integral part both of the country's health system, of which it is the nucleus, and of the overall social and economic development of the community. It is the backbone of the Health for All concept of WHO.

Sn: PHC

Cf. Alma-Ata, secondary health care, tertiary health care

Primary prevention Health: Actions directed towards preventing the initial occurrence of a disease or disorder – WHO.

Society: Laws and actions directed towards preventing the initial breach of laws, order and peace.

Principle of non-refoulement The international principle according to which a person seeking asylum must not be subjected to such administrative measures as refusal of admission at a frontier post or, if he is already in the country, should not be expulsed or obligatorily returned to a country where he might be in danger. This principle is fundamental to the work of UNHCR.

Prion Acronymic word for protein virion. A relatively recently described and not yet fully understood infectious particle composed entirely of protein. It is resistant to known inactivating agents and is implicated in such neuropathological conditions as Alzheimer's and Creutzfeldt-Jakob disease in humans, bovine spongiform encephalitis in cows, scrapie in sheep and similar encephalopathies.
Cf. Creutzfeldt-Jakob disease, mad cow disease, b.s.e., zoonosis

PRISM Acronym for Prognostic Risk of Mortality, a diagnostic scoring system in paediatric critical care medicine based on an index that assesses 34 physiological variables on a severity scale of 1–5.

Prisoner Person deprived of liberty and restricted in activity by the use of force. National and international laws define the extent of a prisoner's restrictions.
Cf. torture

Prisoner of conscience Person imprisoned solely because of his/her political or religious beliefs, gender or racial or ethnic origin, and who has neither used nor advocated violence – AI.

Cf. Amnesty International, torture, Universal Declaration of Human Rights

Prisoner of war A member of the armed forces of a party to conflict, all members of armed groups and units which are under a command responsible to that party and who have been caught and made prisoner by the opposing party in the conflict. Prisoners of war have rights and responsibilities defined by the Geneva Conventions. Guerrillas also benefit from POW provisions.
Sn: POW
Cf. armed conflict, Geneva Conventions, ICRC

Privacy Act A governmental law protecting the privacy of every citizen. In particular, in the United States, the Privacy Act of 1974 upholds the citizens' fundamental right against the misuse of governmental information. In essence, this personal right overrides the public's right, a good factor but which is not free from creating ancillary legal and democratic complications.

Private military and security company/PMSC A commercial non-military company selling security and support services, such as armed or unarmed guards, protection of persons and assets, demining, security training, anti-piracy and anti-hijacking protection, etc., to a variety of state, industrial or private clients, as a business.
Cf. mercenary, UN civilian police, Montreux Document

Privilege Right, exceptional advantage or other benefit belonging to or acquired by a person, a class or office in virtue of their contribution or position, e.g. physician, schoolteacher, school, church, diplomat, member of parliament, the parliament building.

Pro bono More exactly *pro bono publico*, Latin term meaning "for the public good". Voluntary and unpaid service or work undertaken by a person or organization as a humanitarian, altruistic public contribution. Also pro Deo.

Pro-poor health approach An organizational process that stresses the importance of protecting, promoting and improving the health and health conditions of poor people and thereby strengthening development. It constitutes one of the goals within the MDGs.
Cf. poverty, least developed countries, Millennium Development Goals

Probability A measure lying between 0 and 1 which concerns the likelihood that an event is true or will occur, 0 being that the event will not occur.

Probability of damage/of disaster Cf. damage probability formula

Probe Physical: Measuring instrument used in situ and in continuity. Example: probe to measure depth, salinity, temperature.
Medicine: Similar instrument to examine a fistula, deep ulcer.

Processing centre (refugee) A centre where refugees who have been accepted for settlement in a third country live while awaiting their final departure. The term "camp" is not used at UNHCR.
Cf. refugee

Productivity The ratio between the quantity of goods and services produced and the factors that determine it. It is taken as a measure of efficiency.

Prognostic risk of mortality Cf. PRISM

Protection of refugees Cf. refugee protection

Protective food Food of special value which promotes physical development and protects health by virtue of its richness in essential nutrients.
Cf. food fortification, fortified food

Protein The natural nitrogenous substances which, by hydrolysis, give amino acids and constitute an essential factor in cells for the vital functions, growth and repair of all living organisms. Deficiency in protein causes disease.
Cf. protective food

Protein-calorie malnutrition A diversity of pathological conditions arising from coincident shortage or lack of proteins and calories, most frequently occurring in infants and young children and commonly associated with infections.
Sn: protein energy malnutrition.
Cf. malnutrition

Protocol refugee Person who fulfils the definition of refugee according to article I (2) of the Protocol on the status of refugees.
Cf. refugee

Proton Elementary particle carrying positive electrical charge, present in all atoms.
Cf. electron, ionizing radiation

Protrusive dome Type of volcanic dome where the lava has extruded to the surface.
Cf. volcano

Provocation A hostile position, act, threat or aggressiveness, usually uncalled for, expressed by an individual, group, nation or the military, to excite anger, to test opposition or to express dominance.

Pseudomonas Gram-negative bacteria that can produce serious and resistant

infection, especially in immune deficient persons, such as in AIDS or radiation injury.
Cf. immunosuppression

Public health The social and political concept and the health sciences discipline that, at the level of the community or the public, aims at promoting prevention of disease, improving health, prolonging life and enhancing its quality through sanitary living, laws, practices and a healthier environment.
In general, all measures to protect the public's health.
Cf. health, hygiene, primary health care, World Health Organization

Pugwash Conferences on Science and World Affairs Commonly referred to as "Pugwash", a highly regarded international forum named after the town in Canada where eminent scientists and thinkers first met to discuss and propose ways to avoid nuclear war. Since then, conference choices and reflection themes have broadened to include widely different views on social, military, political and international issues, based on impartiality and scientific objectivity. Its deliberations are often heeded by governments, and in 1995, Pugwash and its president jointly received the Nobel Peace Prize.
Cf. WHOPAX Report, Nobel Prize

Purchasing power Ability of individuals or a community to acquire services and goods in function of their income and the prices asked.

Pyroclastic flow In a volcanic eruption, high-density flow or solid magma fragments and gas advancing downslope at speeds reaching 200 km/h, subdivided into ash flow, nuée ardente, glowing avalanche and pumice.

Cf. ash, ash flow, explosivity index, glowing avalanche, nuée ardente, volcanic eruption

Q

Q fever An acute rickettsial disease with fever, headache and pulmonary complications, acquired by inhalation mainly from domestic animals or through ticks.
Cf. zoonosis

Quake Popular term for earthquake.

Quality-adjusted life expectancy (QALE) A model of judgement in which a disability or disease is considered as a factor of reduced quality of life in calculating life expectancy.
Cf. QALY

Quality-adjusted life years (QALY) A measure of adjusting life expectancy by taking into account disabilities, illnesses, handicaps, etc.

Quality health care Cf. medical care quality

Quarantine
1. Obligatory isolation during a given period, prescribed by international law, of a person carrying or coming from an epidemic area with certain specific "quarantinable" communicable diseases.
2. Isolation imposed on ships or aeroplanes coming from infected areas. Cholera, plague and yellow fever are the internationally quarantinable diseases.
Cf. communicable diseases, epidemic

Quicksand Sandy earth which, when saturated and under the influence of hydrostatic pressures, becomes weak, buoyant, unable to bear weight, and tends to flow.
Cf. earth flow

Quinine The classical antimalarial medication and febrifuge. From the alkaloid in cinchona bark, usually taken in sulphate form.

Cf. malaria, mefloquine

R

Rabies A very serious disease due to a virus, common in dogs, foxes, bats but uncommon in man, transmitted by accidental animal bite or contact with its saliva. Death usually ensues due to meningoencephalitis.

Cf. zoonosis, neglected tropical disease

Race A group of people or animals that differs from others in certain visible or invisible characteristics and in the relative frequency of a gene or genes. In reference to populations, it is also used for a community or group of people sharing the same ancestry. Racial discrimination is not tolerable.

Cf. racism

Racism Overt or covert animosity and discrimination against a person, group or population because of race. It is unacceptable according to the Universal Declaration of Human Rights.

Cf. race, human rights

Racketeering Obtaining money, influence or other favours by black-mail, intimidation, force or other illegal means. Destitute persons, disaster stricken people and helpless refugees are often common prey.

Cf. mafia

Rad The old unit of radioactive absorbed dose, equal to one-hundredth of 1 Gy, the SI unit that has replaced it.

Cf. gray, Gy

Radar Acronymic term for Radio Detection and Ranging. A radioelectric method of determining from a single station the direction, distance and speed of an object.

Radiation absorption The ionizing energy absorbed by an exposed population – patient, laboratory worker, explosion victim – from the decay of a radionuclide. The measuring unit is the gray (Gy)

Cf. radiation protection, radiation exposure, gray, sievert

Radiation detriment The detriment of radiation to an exposed population is defined as the mathematical expectation of the harm incurred from an exposure to radiation, taking into account not only the probability of each type of deleterious effect but also the severity of the effects – ICRP.

Cf. radiation exposure, radiation injury, radiation toxicity, radioactive contamination, fallout

Radiation Emergency Medical Preparedness and Assistance Network/REMPAN Better known by its acronym REMPAN, the WHO-led network of over 40 specialized institutions in radiation emergency and public health interventions and long-term follow-up of victims.

Cf. radiation protection, radioactive contamination

Radiation exposure risks/mSv A dose of 100 mSv (millisieverts) results in risk of cancer; 20 mSv is the maximum annual dose allowable for nuclear workers; 10 mSv is the dose received at a whole body scan; 1 mSv is the annual tolerated dose for a person; 0.1 mSv is the dose received at thoracic X-ray examination.

Cf. sievert, radiation detriment, radiation toxicity

Radiation injury Somatic and genetic damage to living organisms caused by ionizing radiation.

Cf. immunodeficiency, ionizing radiation

Radiation protection The measures taken in order to ensure the protection of man and his environment against the consequences of ionizing radiation.
Cf. ionizing radiation, Lugol's iodine, maximum acceptable dose, radioactive decontamination

Radiation sickness Severe nausea, vomiting, lethargy are some of the earliest symptoms of acute radiation exposure, as seen after the Hiroshima nuclear bombing.
Sn: acute radiation syndrome
Cf. Hiroshima/Nagasaki, Chernobyl, Fukushima

Radiation toxicity Toxicity and harmful effects due to radioactivity from a radionuclide present in the body.
Cf. radioactive contamination, sievert, technological disaster

Radioactive cloud Sn: nuclear cloud
Cf. fallout

Radioactive contamination The undesirable presence of radioactive material in the air, in men, in the soil, water, food or on any substance.
Cf. radioactivity, contamination, Chernobyl, radiation detriment

Radioactive decontamination Measures taken to eliminate or reduce the radioactive contamination or pollution of a body, surface, soil or environment.
Cf. radioactive contamination

Radioactive fallout Sn: nuclear fallout
Cf. fallout

Radioactive half-life In the process of diminishing activity of a radioactive substance, the time necessary for half the number of radionuclides to disintegrate.
Sn: half-life
Cf. radioactivity

Radioactive iodine Cf. Iodine-131

Radioactive waste Used material which is contaminated or contains radionuclides at concentrations higher than clearance levels and which will not be reused.
Cf. nuclear waste, Sellafield, La Hague, Windscale

Radioactivity The phenomenon of spontaneous disintegration in a nuclide accompanied by the emission of ionizing radiation.
Cf. nuclear activity, ionizing radiation

Radio astronomy Study of the natural radioelectric rays of cosmic origin.

Radionuclide Species of atom characterized by the number of protons and of neutrons in its nucleus, with properties of spontaneous disintegration. Usually specified by the symbol of the element and the mass number, as in 235U or uranium-235 and cesium-137.
Cf. radionuclide maximum acceptable concentration

Radionuclide maximum acceptable concentration The radioactivity of a nuclide in the air or in drinking water which, when inhaled or ingested, produces the maximum admissible dose in the receiver.
Cf. radionuclide

Radium A radioactive metallic alkaline element of the earth, used in medical therapy. Half-life 1,620 years. Symbol Ra.
Cf. radioactivity, radioactive half-life

Radon A zero-valent radioactive element of short half-life (3.82 days) formed by the disintegration of radium. Directly inserted radon "seeds" are used in cancer therapy.

Rainfall amount The measure of the total amount of liquid precipitation in a given place and time.
Sn: pluviometry
Cf. precipitation, cyclonic rain

Rainout The washing out, by concurrent rain, of the radioactivity from the mushroom cloud produced by nuclear explosion. The oncoming rain may in fact be induced by the heat of the explosion itself.
Sn: washout
Cf. scavenging, mushroom cloud

Rainy season Term used mainly in tropical regions for the annually recurring period of high rainfall which is preceded and followed by dry periods. In the latitudes concerned, this season is often the cause of flood disasters.
Cf. tropical climate, macroclimate

Raison d'état French diplomatic term meaning "Reason of State". According to this political doctrine, a State's interests or well-being override moral, military or other considerations.

Rapid assessment protocol/RAP A brief but valid evaluation, usually with established checklist, to assess the emergency needs of a disaster-affected community in health, survival necessities and services.
Cf. assessment/disaster

Rapprochement A French term, much used in social and diplomatic relations, that refers to gradual normalization and reestablishment of relations after a period of cooling, conflict or disharmony.

Ratification A State's formal approval of a Treaty, by which it officially becomes a state party and has to abide by the stipulations and requirements of that treaty.

Ration (food) Fixed quantity of a specific food or combination of foods provided or distributed to certain individuals or categories of persons, e.g. the army, or to entire populations in special circumstances, as in times of food shortage, war, refugees or disaster.
Cf. emergency feeding, food relief, food shortage

Reactor Sn: nuclear reactor, atomic reactor

Realizing Rights: The Ethical Globalization Initiative Founded by former President of Ireland and High Commissioner for Human Rights, Mary Robinson, this NGO proposes and strives for an ethical foundation to globalization, the need for a new global order built on respect of human rights and understanding between peoples.
Cf. Universal Declaration of Human Rights

Reanimatology Syn: resuscitology
Cf. resuscitation

Recession Marine: ebb.
Finance: slump in trade.
Biology: Mendelian genetic recessive trait.

Recipient Person, group, nation or country that is the beneficiary of aid or technical assistance to meet particular needs, emergency or otherwise.
Sn: donee, beneficiary
Cf. international aid, technical assistance

Recognized refugee Person who is formally recognized as a refugee by the authorities of a State that has signed the international instruments relative to the status of refugees.
Cf. refugee

Reconstruction The phase that follows a disaster, consisting of reorganization of the stricken territory, the restructuring of the built environment and the development of the economy, with the view to re-establishing the pre-disaster conditions.

Cf. rehabilitation

Recovery The restoration, and improvement where appropriate, of facilities, livelihoods and living conditions of the disaster-affected communities, including efforts to reduce further disaster risk factors – UNISDR.

Cf. reconstruction, rehabilitation

Red Crescent The counterpart of the Red Cross in Islamic countries.

Cf. Red Cross

Red Cross Red Cross, or International Red Cross, general terms used for one or all the components of the worldwide organization active in humanitarian work. The official overall name is the International Red Cross and Red Crescent Movement, which has three components.

1. International Committee of the Red Cross (ICRC): acts mainly in conflict disasters as neutral intermediary in hostilities and for the protection of war victims. Guardian of the Geneva Conventions and of International Humanitarian Law.

2. International Federation of Red Cross and Red Crescent Societies (IFRC): federation of all the National Societies, active in non-conflict disasters and natural calamities humanitarian aid.

3. The individual National Red Cross or Red Crescent Society of every country.

Red Cross Principles The seven Fundamental Principles of the Red Cross and Red Crescent Movement are humanity, impartiality, neutrality, independence, voluntary service, unity, universality.

Red Cross symbols The three official symbols of the Red Cross and Red Crescent Movement are the Red Cross, the Red Crescent and the Red Diamond.

Red Diamond The recently introduced symbol, counterpart of the Red Cross in Israel.

Cf. Red Cross symbols

Redevelopment Extensive reorganization of a given area with the view to meeting the needs of the population concerned, by providing the necessary facilities and making better use of the available resources.

Cf. need, resources

Refoulement Expulsion of a refugee towards his country. Such action is reprehensible to the international community. The principle of non-refoulement.

Sn: expulsion

Cf. international community, principle of non-refoulement

Refugee A person who is outside his country of origin and who, due to well-founded fear of persecution, is unable or unwilling to avail himself of that country's protection – UNHCR.

There are different categories of refugees, as given below:

Cf. Convention refugee
de facto refugee
de jure refugee
economic refugee
environmental refugee
internal refugee
mandate refugee
Protocol refugee
recognized refugee
refugee sur place
statutory refugee.

UN High Commissioner for Refugees

Refugees International Important independent NGO active in advocacy, assistance and protection issues of refugees, stateless persons and displaced populations
Cf. refugee, stateless, migration, UNHCR

Refugee processing centre Cf. processing centre

Refugee protection International protection of refugees and displaced persons outside their country and who do not enjoy the protection of their country of origin. Such protection accorded by the High Commissioner for Refugees is based on the 1951 Convention and 1967 Protocol of the UN, the Convention and Protocols of the International Red Cross and on such regional instruments as the 1969 Convention of the Organization of African Unity.
Cf. United Nations High Commissioner for Refugees, principle of non-refoulement, refugee, Geneva Conventions, international protection

Refugee sur place Person who, while not being a refugee when he left his country, becomes one as a result of intervening circumstances.
Cf. refugee

Rehabilitation The operations and decisions after a disaster, with the view to restoring to the stricken country, communities, families and individuals the former living conditions while at the same time encouraging and facilitating the necessary adjustments to the changes caused by the disaster to ensure development.
Cf. adaptation, reconstruction

Rejection Not accepting, not believing, refusing, denying.
Psychology: Denial, in certain circumstances not accepting the evident, e.g. that a parent has died or that a disaster has hit. May be used as a protective mechanism to avoid reality.
Law: The denial, against all evidence, by a powerful person or autocratic ruler, of all wrongdoing. Impunity.
Cf. denial, impunity

Relative risk (disease) The ratio of the incidence of a given disease in exposed or at-risk persons, to the incidence of that disease in unexposed persons.

Reliability The probability that a structure, device, method or system will operate without failure under given conditions for a specific period of time.
Cf. failure

Relief Assistance in material facilities, personal needs and services given to needy persons or communities, without which they would suffer.
Cf. aid, emergency relief, international assistance

Religious sects All major religions have movements of belief and practice that have evolved out of the mainstream teachings of orthodoxy and which have implications on health, medical care, society, the law and human rights. Examples: Jehovah's Witnesses, Scientology, Amish Order, etc.

Rem Acronym for Roentgen Equivalent Man. Previously a unit of ionizing radiation that causes the same damage to humans as 1 roentgen of X-rays, now replaced by Sv, sievert (1 Sv = 100 rem)

Remote sensing The study, exploration and observation of a faraway area, phenomenon or object in space by distant study through satellite-provided data.
Cf. remote sounding

Remote sounding The methodical local exploration of a given environment or unattainable point (e.g. beneath a

collapsed building) carried out from a distance by the use of signals.
Cf. remote sensing

Repatriation The actions and measures taken to ensure the return of a person to his country of origin or of usual residence.
Cf. voluntary repatriation

Representative The delegate of an international organization to a country or to another organization. Organizations have different names for their representatives, e.g. delegate (ICRC), resident representative (UNDP), programme coordinator (WHO), cooperant (France), expert

Request for disaster assistance Official approach made by the authorities of a disaster-stricken country to other governments, international organizations or voluntary agencies requesting aid in face of the calamity.
Cf. declaration of disaster

Rescue Immediate assistance to a person who is injured, e.g. fracture, or in distress, e.g. trapped in a collapsed building, with the view to applying first aid and delivering him from harm.
Cf. first aid

Reservoir of infection Any physical, animal, plant or human source harbouring and favouring the development of pathogens susceptible to be transmitted to man or animals.
Cf. carrier, infection, transmission

Resettlement Relocation and more or less orderly settlement, for temporary or permanent habitation, of refugees and other persons displaced from their usual place of residence.
Cf. displaced person, crisis relocation, refugee, settlement

Residence time The average length of time during which pollutants, such as smoke, toxic chemicals, radioactivity, remain in the atmosphere from the time the pollution begins.
Cf. atmospheric pollution, Chernobyl, Seveso, superfire

Resilience A given person's, community's, or society's capacity to learn from, adapt to, and resist a real or potential hazard (such as a volcano or adverse indoctrination), contain its effects, proceed to recovery and maintain acceptable levels of ordinary living and functioning.
Cf. adaptability, coping capacity

Resource planning and development Study and application of legislative, economic, financial and planning measures to promote a harmonious equilibrium among the activities, the amenities, the population needs and the country's resources over the national territory.
Cf. resources, natural resources management, sustainable development

Respiratory distress syndrome (Acute) A condition of acute pulmonary inflammation with respiratory insufficiency and lack of arterial oxygen, due, among other causes, to multiple trauma and crush injuries.
Cf. asphyxia, dyspnoea
Sn: ARDS
Cf. SARS

Resuscitation/Resuscitology The scientific techniques and manoeuvres applied to reverse acute terminal states and reanimate victims in clinical death, by using intensive care and intensive therapy methods.
The discipline is called resuscitology or reanimatology – after Safar.

Retained dose Following exposure to a given pollutant, the portion of the absorbed dose that persists in the individual after a given time.
Cf. absorbed dose

Retrofitting Strengthening and structurally upgrading existing buildings (houses, dams, bridges, etc.) to withstand destructive forces such as earthquakes and floods and to bring them closer to acceptable construction standards. Rehabilitating a weak structure.

Retrograde amnesia A type of memory loss, of varying length of time, that often follows head injury, with loss of memory for events leading up to the accident.
Cf. amnesia

Retrovirus A pathogenic virus of higher organisms with RNA genome that has the ability to insert a DNA copy of its genome into the chromosome of the host.

Returnee Person who, after having crossed an international boundary as a refugee, returns voluntarily to his country of origin or of usual residence. (Term used by the HCR).
Cf. refugee, voluntary repatriation

Richter scale Logarithmic scale, −1 to 8, indicating the magnitude or "size" of an earthquake, calculated on the amplitude of the seismic waves. All tremors 4, 5 or over are internationally recorded.
– An earthquake of amplitude 3 corresponds to a tremor felt over a limited area.
– 4.5 can cause light destruction.
– 6.6 causes considerable destruction.
– 7–8 causes very great destruction.
– Over 8, total destruction.
Cf. Mercalli scale, earthquake, seismograph, UNESCO

Rickets Disease due to nutritional deficiency in vitamin D. (Not to be confused with rickettsial fevers.)
Sn: hypovitaminosis D
Cf. vitamin deficiency

Rickettsial fever(s) A group of acute diseases characterized by fever and skin eruption due to rickettsiae. Four groups are known: typhus, Rocky Mountain spotted fever, Q fever and trench fever. The agent has been used as a biological weapon.
(Not to be confused with rickets.)
Sn: rickettsial diseases, rickettsiosis
Cf. Q fever, typhus, tick-borne typhus

Ridge Sn: oceanic ridge

Rightagainstdiscrimination Everyone is entitled to the rights and freedoms set forth in the UDHR without any discrimination. Article 2 of the Universal Declaration of Human Rights.
Cf. discrimination, xenophobia, UDHR

Right to a nationality Everyone has the right to belong to a nation. Article 15 of UDHR.
Cf. apatride

Right to assurance of human rights The right to a social order that assures all persons' human rights. Article 28 of UDHR.
Cf. human rights

Right to asylum A persecuted person has the right to asylum in other countries. Article 14 of UDHR.
Cf. asylum, refugee, displaced person

Right to community participation The right to community social life for full development. Article 29, UDHR.
Cf. community, society

Right to cultural participation The right to cultural life in a community. Article 27 of UDHR.
Cf. community, social group

Right to education The right to education. Proclaimed by Article 26 of UDHR.
Cf. Millennium Development Goals

Right to equality All people are equal. Proclaimed by Article 1 of UDHR.
Cf. Universal Declaration of Human Rights, rights fundamental

Right to family privacy The right to freedom from interference with privacy and family. Article 12 of UDHR.
Cf. family unit

Right to free movement Freedom to move in and out of a country. Article 13 of UDHR.

Right to freedom from arbitrary arrest or exile Everyone has the right to be free from arbitrary arrest or exile. Proclaimed by Article 9 of the Universal Declaration of Human Rights.
Cf. human rights, UDHR, displaced person, deportation

Right to freedom from slavery Everyone has the right to be free from slavery. Article 4, UDHR.
Cf. man-induced disaster

Right to freedom from torture Everyone has the right to be free from torture or degrading treatment. Article 5, UDHR.
Cf. torture

Right to freedom of opinion Freedom of opinion and information. Article 19, UDHR.
Cf. democracy

Right to health Right to health, well-being and adequate standard of living. Proclaimed by Article 25 of UDHR and the Constitution of WHO.
Cf. health, World Health Organization, Health for All

Right to intervene By international law, every State has absolute sovereignty over its national territory and its internal affairs, and no outside interference is tolerated. In view, however, of certain unacceptable injustices and totalitarian acts carried out by dictatorial regimes, in 1991, UN Resolution 688 introduced the concept of the right to intervene on humanitarian grounds, e.g. in Iraq. (But so-called "humanitarian war" should never be used as a synonym.) Resolution 43–131 also recognizes the role of NGOs in providing humanitarian aid in "…food, medicine and health care", e.g. in Bosnia-Herzegovina. Subsequent decisions have further codified the concept of the right to intervene, while some even extend this to a duty to intervene.
Sn: droit d'ingérence, R2P, right to protection
Cf. human rights, International Humanitarian Law, international aid, right to protection, sovereignty

Right to life, liberty and security Everyone has the right to life, liberty and personal security. Article 2 of UDHR.

Right to own property Everyone has the right to own property alone, or in association with others. Article 17 of UDHR.

Right to social security Every person has the right to social security. Article 22 of UDHR.

Rights-based development An essential approach to development that describes situations not simply in terms of human needs or of developmental requirements, but in terms of society's obligations to respond to the inalienable rights of individuals, empowers people to demand justice as a right, not as charity, and gives communities a moral basis from which to claim international assistance when needed – K. Annan.
Cf. development, Millennium Development Goals

Rights, inalienable, fundamental The Preamble of the Universal Declaration of Human Rights declares: All human beings are born with equal and inalienable rights and fundamental freedoms.
Cf. Universal Declaration of Human Rights

Rigours Sensation of extreme chill, with severe chattering of teeth, shivers and gooseflesh indicative of lack of adequate body heat. Situation quite frequent in disasters and exposed refugee camps.

Riot-control gases Chemical harassing agents – CN, CS, DM – that are tear gases used for crowd dispersal and riot-armed control. Among the chemical weapons, their use is not prohibited.
Cf. chemical weapons

Rising tide Time interval during which the tide current is directed approximately in the same way as the direction of the sea current.
Sn: flood tide
Cf. tide

Risk Expected loss of lives, persons injured, property damaged and economic activity disrupted, due to a particular hazard for a given area and a reference period. Risk is the product of hazard and vulnerability – UN.
Cf. elements at risk, hazard, vulnerability, acceptable risk, risk management

Risk analysis/assessment The use of available data and information to identify hazards and to estimate the risk – ISO.
Sn: risk assessment
Cf. hazard, risk, risk evaluation

Risk evaluation On the basis of risk analysis, judgement as to whether a risk which is acceptable has been achieved in a given context based on the current values of society – ISO.
Cf. hazard, risk, risk indicator, risk management

Risk indicator Descriptor that briefly denotes a risk that may cause a certain damage or disaster.
Cf. risk map, disaster prevention

Risk management The application of management policies, techniques, methods and practices with the view to analyzing, evaluating, controlling and diminishing risk.
Cf. hazard, risk

Risk map Cartographic representation of the types and degrees of hazard and of natural phenomena that may cause or contribute to a disaster.
Cf. risk indicator, vulnerability study, zoning

Risk reduction–non-structural Besides structural measures to reduce risk, there are non-structural measures that include measures not involving physical construction that uses knowledge, practice or agreement to reduce risks and impacts, in particular through policies and laws, public awareness raising, training and education – UNISDR.
Cf. disaster management, disaster mitigation, risk

Risk transition (health) In the health field, transition that is characterized by such patterns as reduction in infectious disease factors, e.g. undernutrition, unsafe water, poor sanitation, and an increase in risk factors for chronic diseases, e.g. overweight, alcohol abuse, tobacco.
Cf. relative risk

River basin Region drained by a part or all of one or several rivers and their tributaries.
Sn: catchment basin, watershed, hydrological basin, catchment area

River blindness Sn: onchocerciasis

River forecast The expected discharge of a river or stream, especially of the volume of flow, into a reservoir.

Road traffic crash/injury A collision or incident occurring on a public road, involving at least one moving vehicle; a road crash injury that results from a road traffic crash – WHO.

Robben Island Guidelines Reflecting the African Charter on Human and Peoples' Rights, this set of humanitarian and practical guidelines constitutes a further tool for the prevention of torture and the treatment of prisoners.
Cf. torture, Universal Declaration of Human Rights, APT

Rock slide The sudden fall of rock masses and fragments and earth along a slope.
Sn: landslide, mudslide

Rockefeller Foundation Classical benevolent foundation since the beginning of the twentieth century. Active in a wide gamut of health, humanitarian and scientific endeavours. Was instrumental in the founding of the London School of Hygiene and Tropical Medicine and the Peking Union Medical College. It donated the land in New York on which the UN building now stands.

Rocky Mountain spotted fever Cf. rickettsial fever

Rodenticide A toxic chemical compound used for the elimination of rodents.
Cf. pesticide

Roentgen The unit of exposure to radiation.

Roller A form of violent coastal surge with a spiral curling movement of the wave crest.

Roma people A term of Sanskrit origin, meaning man, without any reference to Rome, Romania or Greece. A nomadic people without fixed national status or cultural and historic origin, which tends to stigmatize and marginalize them.
Cf. Tsiganes, nomad, gypsies

Rome Declaration A proposal for a model of aid effectiveness in achieving the Millennium Development Goals and other development results, based on the guidelines for sector-wide approaches (SWAps) to health development.

Rotary International A worldwide organization composed of local and national "Rotarian" members representing professional and business community leaders who provide philanthropic services and funds in all walks of life, promoting goodwill and ethical standards. A worthwhile programme has been the fight for polio eradication.

Royal College of Physicians and Surgeons of Canada The official qualifying body of physicians and surgeons in Canada devoted to maintain high-quality care, research, studies, ethics and surgical specialization. Also promotes proficiency in essential surgery in developing countries and awards its Humanitarian Medal to deserving doctors working in poorer regions.
Cf. essential surgery, CIDA

Rupture zone In seismology, the line of fault breakage corresponding to a particular earthquake sequence.
Cf. fault, fracture

Rural Any area which is predominantly agricultural and farmland, intermingled with forest and vegetation and scattered with residences and other development, situated some distance from cities and not dependent on industry.

Cf. urbanization, rural health

Rural development Study and applications of measures aiming, within a rural setting, at better utilization of natural resources in function of the needs of the population and within the framework of an environmental policy.

Rural economy Branch of economics and administration with emphasis on agricultural activity that studies the mechanisms of agricultural enterprise and the definition of the rural/agricultural sector within the wider economic context.

Cf. urbanization, industrial complex

Rural health The pattern of diseases and the available health care in rural areas under difficult circumstances. Most of the developing countries are serviced by this level of care, less expensive and more relevant to the population, based on the primary health-care concept and health-care centres to provide essential medicine and surgery, obstetrics, mother and child care, vaccinations, basic medicaments and health advice.

Cf. rural, primary health care

S

Safety at sea The international laws and regulations enacted for the security of maritime navigation and the safety of life at sea.

Cf. Law of the Sea, International Maritime Organization

Saffir-Simpson Scale of Cyclones A scale that takes into account wind speed, the minimum pressure in the eye of the cyclone and the resulting damage. Expressed in 5 categories:

Wind speed km/h   Damage

1. 118–153	Minimal
2. 154–177	Moderate
3. 178–209	Extensive
4. 210–249	Extreme
5. 250>	Catastrophic

Cf. hurricane, Beaufort scale, cyclone

Sago A starch extracted from the pith of the sago palm and used as a foodstuff in certain regions.

Sahel Vast area of semi-arid land bordering the Southern Sahara and covering all or part of Mauritania, Mali, Burkina Faso, Niger, Chad, Senegal, Ghana, Cameroon, Nigeria and the Central African Republic. It is particularly subject to drought and desertification, which is also called Sahelization.

Cf. desertification, CILSS, semi-arid land

Sahelian zone Sn: Sahel

Salmonellosis Infection of the gastrointestinal tract caused by germs of the *Salmonella* group. It presents as a variety of diseases, the infection appearing as an acute gastroenteritis, enteric fever or a focal disease with or without septicaemia. It includes typhoid fever.

Cf. diarrhoeal diseases, carrier, food poisoning, typhoid fever

SAMU   Social   International Cf. International Social EMS

Sand whirl Sn: dust whirl

Sanitary engineering The theory, practice and techniques of medical, construction, hydraulic, town planning, waterworks and other principles applied to public health.

Cf. public health

Sanitary improvement Collection, evacuation and disposal, according to hygienic precepts, of rain water, waste water and solid wastes, with or without prior treatment.

Cf. waste water

Sanitation The application of measures and techniques aimed at ensuring and improving environmental health in a community, including the collection, evacuation and disposal of rain and used liquid and solid wastes, with or without prior treatment.

Sn: sanitary improvement

Cf. waste water, water treatment

Sarcophagus In ancient Greece, a stone coffin. In the thermonuclear industry, when a reactor explodes, melts down or fails beyond repair, it is totally cocooned or "mothballed" to prevent further escape of radiation, definitively covered in its entirety with very thick, heavily reinforced concrete, known as sarcophagus. This was done to the exploded reactor in Chernobyl.

Sarin A highly lethal nerve gas, used as a chemical weapon for terrorism or war. Notorious incident at Tokyo railway station in March 1995.

Cf. nerve gas, chemical warfare, terrorism, Geneva Protocol

Sasakawa Foundation Cf. Nippon Foundation

Satellite An object that orbits around a larger one. Artificial satellites orbiting the earth are now used for communications, monitoring weather, gathering hydrological, agricultural, seismological and other similar data and observing environmental phenomena. Also used for military purposes.

Sn: artificial satellite.

Cf. meteosat, probe, space station, World Weather Watch

Savannah Semi-arid region (dryness ratio 1 to 7) of grasslands across which shrubs and trees are scattered. The grasses are typically tall and fast-growing that become dormant during and immediately after the short wet season. For the remainder of the year, they are brown and dry, particularly prone to extensive fire disasters.

Cf. desert, desertification, Sahel, semi-arid zone, vegetation fire

Scabies A highly transmissible parasitic skin infection characterized by intense itching, superficial burrows, especially between the fingers and in the skin folds, and secondary infection due to scratching. Can spread to entire families and communities in crowded conditions. Treatment is effective.

Sn: the itch

Cf. parasitic diseases

Scavenging The removal by precipitation or clouds of radiation particles or gases deposited in the atmosphere following a nuclear explosion.

Cf. rainout

Schistosomiasis A group of parasitic diseases prevalent in endemic form in many areas, caused by flukes *(Schistosoma)* and transmitted through freshwater snails as intermediate hosts.

Sn: bilharzia

Cf. endemic disease, parasitic disease

Scrapie The zoonotic disease of spongiform encephalopathy of sheep, caused by a prion.

Cf. bovine spongiform encephalopathy, prion, zoonosis

Screening The presumptive search for and identification of unrecognized disease, defect or disorder through the application of tests, examinations, questions and other rapid procedures.

Scurvy A severe nutritional disease due to deficiency of vitamin C (ascorbic acid), characterized by bleeding gums, gingivitis, bone pain, swelling over the ends of the long bones and generally poor condition. It is easily preventable by eating citrus fruits and fresh fruits and vegetables.

Sn: hypovitaminosis C, ascorbic acid deficiency

Sea bed In the marine environment, the interface between the solid floor and the liquid overlay.

Sn: sea floor

Cf. estuary, hydrography, littoral

Sea conditions An assessment of the agitation of the surface of the sea. The state of the sea is expressed numerically by the Douglas scale or by the height of the waves.

Sea floor Sn: sea bed

Sea level The actual level of the sea constantly changes; the mean level at a stable place is determined by averaging all the levels over a given period.

Cf. swell, tide, wave

Sea surge A rise in sea level that results in the inundation of coastline areas. These phenomena are caused by the movements of the ocean, sea currents, winds and major storms – OFDA.

Search and rescue/SAR The extensive system using air, sea, land and other means employed to look for, locate, rescue and recover disaster victims and apply the necessary emergency aid and treatment. INSARAG, the International Rescue Advisory Group, coordinates these efforts worldwide.

Cf. first aid, rescue, survival chain, SAR

Season In meteorology, the climatic division of the year into periodic sections, varying according to the latitude. In middle latitudes, the division corresponds to the farming year; in the northern and southern hemisphere, the divisions are autumn, winter, spring, summer. In the tropics, the division into seasons is usually made in terms of rainfall or, in places, of wind direction, thus, in India, dry season or rainy season, or "north-east monsoon" and "south-west monsoon". In the continental subtropical regions, the seasons are usually defined in terms of temperature (cold or hot season) or rainfall (dry or rainy season) or both.

Secondary hazard An emergency or hazard that follows or is caused by another hazard or disaster, e.g. epidemic following famine, fires following an earthquake, landslides after floods, malnutrition after drought, avalanche after volcanic eruption (Nevado del Ruiz), mass blindness after chemical explosion (Bhopal), extensive goitre and cancer after nuclear accident (Chernobyl)

Cf. fallout, hazard

Secondary healthcare facility Diseases that cannot be managed at the peripheral primary health-care level are referred to a secondary health-care facility which is more specialized and can meet more advanced diagnostic and therapeutic needs, such as radiography, general surgery, complicated pregnancy, etc., by trained staff. More complicated and specialized conditions are referred to a tertiary health-care centre.

Cf. tertiary health care, primary health care

Sector-wide approach to health development (SWAp) An important element of the international efforts to harmonize and align development assistance around national policies and strategies. Built on the premise that all significant funding for the sector supports a single sector policy and expenditure programme, under government leadership, adopting common approaches across the sector and progressing towards relying on government procedures to disburse and account for all funds – WHO.

Cf. Rome Declaration, Millennium Development Goals

Seiche A free or standing wave oscillation of the surface of water in an enclosed basin that is initiated by local atmospheric changes, tidal currents or earthquakes – OFDA.

Seism From the Greek earthquake. Relating to, pertaining to, connected with or produced by an earthquake. Seismicity denotes the frequency of earthquakes in a given area.

Sn: earthquake

Cf. seismograph, seismoscope, Richter scale, Mercalli scale

Seismic epicentre Cf. epicentre

Seismic precursor Sn: foreshock

Seismic sea wave Ocean wave caused by undersea earthquakes, volcanoes or land movements. Tsunami.

Cf. earthquake, tsunami, volcano

Seismic sounding Definition of the position of submarine plates by measuring the time interval that separates the emission of seismic signals and their rebound after reflection and/ or refraction in the variable terrain and onto the sounding reflectors.

Cf. seismograph, sliding fault

Seismograph A highly sensitive instrument for recording the time, amplitude and duration of vibratory movements of the ground, especially earthquakes.

Cf. earthquake, Mercalli scale, Richter scale, seismoscope

Seismoscope An instrument which indicates only the occurrence of an earthquake, without permanently recording it as opposed to the seismograph.

Cf. seismograph

Self-immolation Immolation is sacrifice. Committing suicide by self-destruction, usually by fire, in a public place, is a not uncommon way of attracting attention to a cause, ideal or struggle. Examples: Prague, Tunis.

Cf. suicide bomb, kamikaze

Sellafield Nuclear waste reprocessing plant in England built to recycle the unused uranium 235 and plutonium 239 from nuclear industry into fuel for nuclear reactors. Highly controversial due to the risks of very serious radioactive contamination. Suffered five radioactive incidents of INES level 4 in 1955 and 1979.

Cf. nuclear reactor, nuclear waste, radioactive contamination, atom bomb, Windscale, La Hague, Three Mile Island, International Nuclear Event Scale

Semaphore Post or apparatus for sending signals by day or night through a system of oscillating arms, lanterns or flags. Verb to signal. In Italy, it means traffic lights.

Semi-arid zone Zone, bordering an arid region, in which the precipitation is insufficient (dryness ratio 1 to 7) to maintain agriculture and where artificial irrigation is needed if cultivation is to be carried out. Particularly prone to extensive fire disasters.

Cf. desert, desertification, Sahel, savannah

Semi-permanent anticyclone Region where high pressures predominate during about half of the year and where an anticyclone appears on the corresponding seasonal mean pressure chart.

Cf. anticyclone

September 11, 2001 / 9/11 On 11 September 2001, a coordinated series of catastrophic terrorist suicidal attacks using hijacked civilian aircraft smashed against and totally destroyed the Twin Towers of the New York Trade Centre, and partly damaged the Pentagon, causing immense destruction, some 3,000 dead and over 6,000 injured. The worst foreign attack on US soil to date. The American and worldwide responses have caused significant revisions in national and international defence strategies, psychological and political perceptions of peace, alliances, travel regulations, terrorist suppression and subsequent conflicts.

Sn: popularly known as 9/11

Cf. terrorism, man-made disaster

Septic tank A method of static sewage disposal based on water filtrage through an earthen pit, where there is no sewer canalization.

Serum The liquid part of blood plasma that contains all the components of blood except the clotting factor fibrinogen.

Serum hepatitis Cf. viral hepatitis B

Services An activity or its result that is of value to individuals and to society, but which does not consist of economic goods or of tangible products. Examples: public transport, medical service, education, city lighting.

Settlement

1. Introduction, in a given place, of new facilities, such as buildings, factories, schools, according to a plan, called a settlement or development plan.

2. Introduction, in a given site, of a population, where it establishes and develops, according to a resettlement plan.

Severe weather threat An indicator, the severe weather threat index – SWEAT – is used to predict tornadoes and thunderstorms – WMO.

Seveso A village near Milan, Italy, site of a chemical plant which, in July 1976, accidentally discharged the toxic compound dioxin, causing severe illness and toxic manifestations among the surrounding population, with extensive environmental damage. Subject of EU Directive 501/82 which sets regulations and emergency plans for any industrial activity that may be "a major accident hazard".

Cf. dioxin, technological disaster, toxicological disaster

Sewage/Sewerage A community's used water system, carrying washed-up material, domestic, communal and industrial, together with any rain and surface water. The technical aggregate of collecting pipes, conduits and pumping stations is called sewerage. A critical problem in disasters and refugee camps.

Sexual abuse An act forcibly performed by a person of trust and responsibility against a vulnerable person, e.g. a child. It is a criminal act punishable by law.

Sexual harassment Social, psychological or physical pressure exerted by a person of trust, authority or confidence on a weaker person of dependence or lower rank, with the aim of winning sexual favours.

Sexual violence Any unconsented sexual act, or act with sexual connotation, attempt to coerce, provoke or obtain a sexual act or an act to use a person for sexual traffic or exploitation, regardless of the relationship of the persons concerned and in any setting. Any sexual act on a minor.

Cf. violence against women

Sexually transmitted diseases Diseases transmitted by sexual contact constitute the most common communicable diseases in the world. Some are specific, others are non-specific, and include gonorrhoea, syphilis, genital warts, AIDS, urethritis, trichomoniasis, candidiasis, etc.

Sn: venereal disease, STD, VD

Shaman/Shamanism Originally a primitive religion of the Ural-Altaic people of Siberia, in which all good and evil in life is believed to be caused by spirits. Shaman priests or spiritual medicine-men can intervene (e.g. as healers), being the initiated intermediaries between the common people and the unseen world of spirits. – Skil Da Gatkun

Cf. totemism, traditional medicine, aborigine

Shanty town Disorderly conglomeration of improvised dwellings with minimal or absent public services, consisting of unsanitary shacks, constructed with reclaimed materials, often built in and contributing to an unsanitary environment. Called favela in South America.

Cf. slum dwelling, favela

Sharia Arabic term for the body of Islamic law based on the Quran and on the practices undertaken or approved by the Prophet and established as legally binding precedents.

Cf. fatwa

Shear The difference in the velocity of the wind at various altitudes.

Shear wall A structural element that resists lateral forces – UNDRO.

Shelter The necessary, essential physical cover and protection in the form of tents, sheeting, shacks, for disaster victims or displaced persons who have lost access to their normal homes or habitations and who must have some defence against the rain, snow, wind, cold, heat, etc., and maintain some privacy. Food, water, shelter are the main immediate needs of people in disaster. In disaster and refugee situations, the basic requirement is 3.5 sq. metres per person. For a collectivity, 30 sq. m. are needed.

Cf. sheltering, shelter needs, essential bodily needs

Shelter needs Essential covered shelter space needed in disaster situations is $3.5–5.5 \text{ m}^2$ per person depending on climatic conditions.

Cf. shelter, essential bodily needs

Sheltering Action that consists of providing asylum or provisional lodgings to an individual or group.

Shigellosis Cf. bacillary dysentery

Shock Medicine: An acute condition in which the flow of blood to the tissues and the output of the heart are not adequate to sustain the body's normal functions and may lead to death unless emergency measures are taken.

Cf. basic life support, survival chain

Psychology: The extreme degree of stress, panic or anxiety attack that certain individuals may present in an emergency or disaster. See also post-traumatic stress disorder.

Shock wave A critical point in the interface between two waves when the velocity, and consequently the pressure and density, jumps to new values, with the decompression of air at high speeds, and occurring naturally in space or when man-made supersonic objects transverse it – at a speed higher than the speed of sound.

Shore profile The line of the coast formed by the constant accumulating and abrasive action of the waves.

Cf. wave, littoral

Sievert (Sv) Unit of radiation dose. Has replaced the rem (1 Sv = 100 rem).

Symbol Sv. For harmful radiation exposure doses in millisieverts (mSv), see radiation exposure risks.

Siting Cf. settlement

Size of earthquake Vernacular term, the correct designation is magnitude of the earthquake.
Cf. Richter scale

Skimmed milk powder Sn: dried skimmed milk, DSM

Slant distance In nuclear explosion, the distance from a given point on the surface of the earth to a point where the explosion occurs.

Sleeping sickness A chronic, often fatal sickness in tropical Africa transmitted by the tsetse fly. Another variant is common in South America, where it is known as Chagas' disease.
Sn: Chagas' disease, African trypanosomiasis

Sliding fault Subvertical shearing plane along which two plates of lithosphere or two active segments of oceanic ridge slide upon each other.
Sn: transform fault
Cf. earthquake, oceanic ridge, seismic sounding

Slow disaster Disaster, usually natural, the beginnings of which are slow, sometimes imperceptible until the full effect is felt, as in poor crops leading to drought and famine.
Sn: creeping disaster
Cf. disaster, natural disaster, sudden impact disaster

Slum Cf. shanty town, slum dwelling

Slum dwelling Lodgings that, by their poor construction, conditions of occupation, lack of upkeep and siting, do not meet the needs of comfort and sanitation and contribute to social and health deprivation.
Sn: shanty town, slum, favela

Smallpox A highly contagious lethal disease caused by the *vaccinia* group of viruses, transmitted from person to person. It was the first disease for which vaccination was professionally applied (1721) and the first to have been totally eradicated (since 1977) through the programme of WHO.
Sn: variola major and minor
Cf. immunization, vaccination, World Health Organization.

Smoke yield The mass of smoke produced per gram of material burnt.

SMS/GOES Satellites Synchronous Meteorological Satellites/Geostationary Operational Environmental Satellites. Satellites orbiting over the equator at the same rate as the earth's rotation and providing to ground receiving stations images of visible and infrared portions of the spectrum for the same area every 30 min – UNDRO.

Social accountability Society: The responsibility of serving society for the benefit of the population it is derived from.
Health: In the field of health, the social accountability of medical schools can be defined as the obligation to direct education, research and service activities towards addressing the priority health concerns of the country, region and/or nation they have a mandate to serve – WHO.

Social behaviour The aggregate actions and reactions of a person or group when relating to a given social environment and which can be objectively observed.

Social cost The total monetary and communal cost or health burden to society due to any kind of economic activity, e.g. asbestos mining causing long-term pulmonary impairment.

Social group Groups of individuals, within a population, who share one or several characteristics that distinguish them sociologically. Examples: students, retirees, handicapped.

Social indicators Different indices used for the assessment of the socio-economic situation of a society. Examples: infantile mortality rates, green spaces per inhabitant, density of motor traffic, literacy rates.
Cf. society

Social media/Social network A recent worldwide development in electronic social networking whereby an online service, web or site focuses on establishing social data and links among people who share common interests or activities and who interact via the Internet, Tweeter, Facebook or similar media. Such quick independent and personal communications can be of great importance in emergencies, as was the case in the 2011 Arab uprisings. It can also be used for harmful purposes.

Societal functions in disasters Disasters are liable to disrupt most basic social facilities and societal functions. For details Cf. basic societal functions.

Society The complex organization of a population group sharing a common culture, institutional resources and obeying common laws. A natural disaster that does not hit man and his society remains a mere geological or meteorological phenomenon.

Society for International Development/SID Explores and promotes dialogue and searches for alternative paths of social transformation for sustainable and just development. Partner in health with WHO.

Society for Medical Care of Chemical War Victims A medical and social organization in Tehran for the immediate and subsequent care of victims of chemical weapons used in the 1987 Iran-Iraq war.
Cf. chemical weapons

Socio-economic survey Enquiry based on social and economic factors, comprising the structure of the family, social attitudes, cultural activities, profession, regular or seasonal employment, revenue, spending power, level of education, size of enterprise, agriculture, etc.
Cf. social indicators

Soil The superficial loose covering of the earth's crust, composed of the breakdown, from weathering, of the bedrock and of the decomposition of organic matter under the physical, chemical and biological action of the environment.

Soil erosion Degradation of the soil through carrying away by wind or water of soil necessary for the forests, food and agriculture. Often caused by mismanagement of the land – a natural and man-made disaster.
Cf. desertification, anthropic erosion

Soil-transmitted helminthiasis Intestinal worm infections found worldwide under poor conditions that in children cause anaemia, stunted growth, avitaminosis A, malnutrition. A neglected disease.
Cf. helminthiasis

Solfatara A vent in a volcano from which only gases are emitted.
Cf. volcano

Somatic cells All cells of the body other than germ cells.

Sorghum Common tropical cereal plant grown for grain and fodder.

Source Emergence of underground water at a point on the surface of the ground.
Sn: spring

Source of infection Any organism, substance, material or object which transmits an infectious agent to a host.
Cf. communicable disease, infection

Sovereignty The primary characteristic of a State which is subordinate to no other State is equal to all others within the United Nations and enjoys authority within its borders and total independence recognized by all States.
Cf. United Nations, right to intervene

Soya-fortified bulghur Food mixture consisting of:
85% bulghur wheat, cracked
15% soya grits, defatted, toasted
Sn: SFB
Cf. food mixtures, bulghur

Soya-fortified cornmeal Food mixture consisting of:
85% cornmeal, degermed
15% soya grits, defatted, toasted.
Sn: SFCM
Cf. food mixtures

Soya-fortified sorghum grits Sorghum preparation enriched with soya, used for supplementary feeding.
Sn: SFSG
Cf. food mixtures, sorghum, supplementary feeding

Space débris The remains of missiles, spacecraft, space exploration stations, probes and military devices left in space after their use or still in operation, presenting an increasing space hazard.
Cf. arsenalization of space

Space probe Uninhabited device for the exploration of space beyond the earth's gravity.
Cf. probe, satellite, World Meteorological Organization

Space station Satellite that does not have its autonomous means of propulsion (or has limited such capacity), placed in space to ensure a mission of a certain length of time.

Cf. satellite

Sphere Project, The The programme of the Steering Committee for Humanitarian Response, launched in 1997, which has developed the Humanitarian Charter, a set of universal minimum standards and indicators for effective assistance in humanitarian disaster response, published as a useful guide.
Cf. International Association for Humanitarian Medicine, Humanitarian Charter, emergency health kit of WHO, standards, indicators

Spill Sn: overspill

Spitak earthquake 1988 The strongest earthquake in the region since historical times, in spite of this Caucasian zone being known as seismic. On 7 December 1988, the Spitak region of Armenia (then in the Soviet Union) was hit disastrously, over 25,000 dead, the city completely destroyed, particularly due to poor construction and bad infrastructure. Outpouring of international solidarity: 111 nations provided aid, and despite Cold War animosity, the Soviet Union exceptionally asked for US assistance, the first since the end of World War II. The new Republic of Armenia still not fully recovered.
Cf. earthquake, FAR

Spontaneous combustion Catching fire from self-heating, as in natural wildfires, without any outside source of heat being applied.

Spring Sn: source

Squall A sudden strong wind of short duration that stands out of the mean velocity of its mainstream.
Sn: gust

Stampede An irrational rush of flight of a group in panic, with risk of trampling, crush and asphyxiation.
Cf. panic

Standard of living The aggregate of goods and services available or accessible to an individual, group or nation, depending on its purchasing power.
Cf. purchasing power

Standards/Indicators In humanitarian assistance, standards are the minimum level to be attained to meet the needs of life with dignity, while indicators are signals that show whether such standards have been attained – Sphere Project.
Cf. Sphere Project

Staple food The most commonly or regularly eaten food in a country or community and which forms the mainstay of the total calorie supply, especially in the poorer populations and at times of food shortage. When referring to staple food, the actual food product must be mentioned.
Cf. conventional food, food

Star wars Sn: Strategic defences initiative
Cf. cyberwar

Starvation The state resulting from extreme privation of food or of drastic reduction in food intake over a long period of time, leading to severe physiological, functional, behavioural, clinical and morphological disturbances.
Cf. famine, slow disaster, undernutrition

Stateless A person who is not officially recognized to have formal, statutory identity with a State, a country or nationality. May be due to expulsion from the country, non-issuance of nationality documents or passport by a conquering power, to discrimination, depriving one of his citizenship, or more rarely, upon voluntary exile, relinquishing or refusal. This is a grave situation in an interdependent world. According to Article 15 of the UDHR, everyone has the right to a nationality and the right to not being arbitrarily deprived of it.
Cf. Universal Declaration of Human Rights, Nansen passport, refugee, displaced person, apatride

Statutory refugee Person recognized as a refugee according to the international accords prior to the 1951 Convention on the status of refugees, as defined by Article I.A of that Convention.
Sn: de jure refugee
Cf. refuge

Sterilization
1. Technique(s) aiming at destroying all living microorganisms.
2. Operation or technique aiming at preventing the reproduction of living organisms.
3. Disinfection.
Cf. decontamination

Sternal punch A manoeuvre in emergency cardiac resuscitation, when the person is pulseless. It consists of delivering a controlled blow with the clenched fist to the base of the sternum. If not successful, it must be followed by external cardiac massage.

Stigma An unjustified negative imputation to a person's or community's reputation or racial characteristics, a shame or a stain of disgrace, closely leading to discrimination and racism.
Cf. discrimination, race, facies

Stochastic modelling A method of modelling which includes elements of probability or chance. In mathematics, stochastic means pertaining to random variables.
Cf. damage probability

Stockholm International Peace Research Institute/SIPRI Very important Swedish institution for studying peace mechanisms, promoting peace, facilitating arbitration, providing peace personnel for the UN and promoting international understanding.

Stockholm syndrome A personal psychological reconditioning through which, after initial aversion and animosity, a victim or detainee develops compassion, loyalty or even love towards his/her captor or prison guard.

Stockpile

1. To store.
2. A place or storehouse where material, medicines and other supplies needed in disaster are kept under good conditions for emergency relief. Example: UN warehouse in Italy, UNIPAC in Copenhagen.
3. In an arms race, the accumulation and storing of nuclear weapons.
4. The stored supplies.

Cf. emergency supplies, supplies

Storm Strong wind with a speed of 44–50 knots. (Force 10 on the Beaufort scale).

The atmospheric disturbance can range from a tornado (1 km across) to tropical cyclones (2,000–3,000 km across).

Cf. Beaufort scale, wind

Storm surge A sudden and often catastrophic rise in the level of the sea as a result of a combination of high winds and low atmospheric pressure.

Cf. tidal wave, storm wave

Storm warning Meteorological message intended to warn those concerned of the actual or expected occurrence of high winds, of Beaufort force 10 or 11, over a specified area.

Cf. cyclone warning, gale warning, hurricane warning, typhoon warning

Strategic Arms Limitation and Reduction Treaty (START) Originally a treaty (START I) negotiated during the Cold War with the aim of reducing the strategic nuclear arms stockpiles of the superpowers, signed in

1991. Subsequently renegotiated between the United States and Russia, START-II came into force on 5 February 2011, each pledging to lower their ceiling of 2,200 nuclear strategic warheads to 1,550 and the nuclear ballistic missiles to 700. The inspection mechanisms remain as those of 1991.

Cf. Strategic defence initiative, Non-Proliferation Treaty, Strategic Arms Limitation Treaty – SALT.

Strategic Arms Limitation Treaty (SALT) Negotiations on the limitation of strategic nuclear arms, signed in 1972, but not ratified.

Cf. Strategic Arms Reduction Treaty – START.

Strategic Defences Initiative The space-based system of nuclear weaponry proposed by the United States as a national defensive initiative. Popularly known as Star Wars.

Cf. arms race, cyberwar, START, anti-missile shield, arsenalization of space

Stratosphere The zone of atmospheric air, above the troposphere, between 10 and 50 km altitude, in which the temperature changes very little with height.

Cf. atmosphere

Stratovolcano Volcanic complex composed of the piling up of lava flows and of pyroclastic beds.

Cf. lava flow, volcano

Stratus cloud

1. A low cloud varying in altitude, between 0 and 2,000 m.
2. A generally grey cloud layer, with uniform base, which may give drizzle, ice or snow.

Stress Health: Any strain, anxiety, psychological shock or excessive pressure that disturbs the smooth functioning of a person or organism (and by extension of a group). Disasters are stressful events.

Cf. panic, post-traumatic stress disorder

Physiology: The normal response of the body to increased demands.

Physics: The force per unit area acting on a material and causing a change in its dimension. Strain.

Stripping Sn: denudation

Stupor Marked diminution or absence of voluntary movements or response to external stimuli, the person being neither unconscious nor asleep. Dissociative stupor is a form caused by a recent stressful event, such as a disaster, or destabilizing social problem.

Cf. post-traumatic stress disorder, panic, shock

Stuxnet The name of a secret military informatics computer virus that can disable military installations. In 2010, it invaded and seriously damaged the computerized uranium enriching centrifuge system at the Nantaz nuclear facility.

Cf. cyberwar, hacking, virus

Subsidence Collapse of a land surface area due to underlying removal of earth or overmining.

Subtropical anticyclone Anticyclone of the subtropical high pressure regions.

Cf. anticyclone

Sudden-impact natural disaster A natural disaster of unexpected (e.g. earthquake) or very quick onset (e.g. cyclone) that usually causes many injuries and deaths, extensive environmental damage and socio-economic upheaval, necessitating major immediate response. Such sudden-impact emergencies may be triggered by earthquakes, cyclones, hurricanes, tornadoes, tsunamis, snowstorms,

blizzards, avalanches, landslides, flash floods, fires, volcanic eruptions.

(The opposite would be a slow-impact, creeping disaster, e.g. drought leading to famine.)

Cf. natural disaster, slow disaster

Suicide bomber/Suicide attack A person who, for any special reason, causes or ideal carries out an attack directly against a chosen target, using oneself as the explosive medium by carrying the bomb, grenade or other explosive device dissimulated on the body and dying in the explosion thus created.

Cf. self-immolation, kamikaze

Summer monsoon Monsoon of oceanic origin that blows in the summer.

Cf. winter monsoon

Superfire The result of merging firestorms and conflagrations caused by the phenomena created by the explosion of a nuclear weapon.

Cf. conflagration, firestorm, nuclear war, catastrophic fires

Supplementary feeding programme/ SFP Programme that aims at correcting nutritional deficiencies by providing certain population groups with nutrients and appropriate meals or snacks, served in addition to their regular meals. This service is usually free or at low cost.

Cf. food aid, food mixtures

Supplies Cf. stockpile, SUMA

Surface water Water flowing or stagnating on the surface of the ground.

Surge Cf. wave

Surgeons OverSeas/SOS SOS is the operational programme of the Society of Humanitarian Surgeons, New York, an NGO of surgeons who carry out training and surgical operations in developing and poor countries on a voluntary, humanitarian basis.

Cf. essential surgery

Surgical conditions Conditions that include any pathology for which an externally applied invasive procedure may provide treatment, cure or palliation. Some conditions may not require incision, e.g. setting of a fracture, and modern techniques are becoming increasingly non-invasive. In poorer countries, at least the services of essential surgery must be provided within primary health care.

Surveillance System that permits the continuous observation, measurement and evaluation of the progress of a process or phenomenon with the view to taking corrective measures. Example: surveillance of the water quality of a river, of air pollution, of health or a cardiac patient.

Sn: monitoring

Survival chain In emergency and critical medicine, the four links in the chain essential for the survival of the victim are (1) early access, to get help, immediate response and call for EMS; (2) early CPR to buy time; cardiopulmonary resuscitation to keep oxygenated blood flowing to the brain until additional help arrives; (3) early defibrillation, to "restart" the heart with an automatic defibrillator and (4) early ACLS, providing advanced cardiac life support with airway clearance, lung ventilation cardiac therapy and necessary monitoring – Laerdal.

Cf. advanced cardiac life support, cardiopulmonary resuscitation, emergency medical services, lifelines, defibrillator

Susceptible case Person vulnerable to infection or other disease.

Sn: vulnerable person

Suspect case A case or person whose medical history or symptoms suggest that he may have, or may be developing or carrying, an infection.

Cf. carrier, incubation period

Sustainable development Development which meets the needs of the present without compromising the ability of future generations to meet their own needs – WCED.

Decisions, processes and actions that meet present needs without creating undue burden to society or the environment and without undermining the ability of coming generations to meet and sustain their own needs.

Cf. development, economic development, primary health care, health, WCED, MDG

Sustainable elimination Industrial products and material developments require that all such improvements and sustainability must also foresee and contain an inbuilt mechanism to ensure the elimination of such material at the end of its productive span, without causing damage to the environment and without harm to the population in the current and subsequent years. The nuclear industry, for instance, cannot guarantee such elimination and therefore falls short of the needed safety imperative.

Cf. sustainable development, nuclear safety, Chernobyl, Fukushima

Swedish International Development Authority/SIDA Commonly known by its acronym SIDA, very important governmental department for international aid for development and in disasters, humanitarian support and cooperation with UN agencies. (Not to confuse with CIDA.)

Swell In a catchment area or watershed, the swelling of a stream or water course to levels above normal, following heavy precipitation and snow thaw.

Cf. catchment area

Swiss Aid/Swissaid Formally the Swiss Agency for Development and Cooperation (SDC), important government-based humanitarian and development organization that provides significant aid in disasters and supports and promotes humanitarian action in a variety of ways.

Synergism The cumulative interaction of several factors resulting in a combined effect that becomes greater than the sum of the separate individual effects. Example: malnutrition, plus pregnancy, plus cold temperature have an aggregate effect which is more serious than any of the three conditions separately. Similarly with compound disasters.

Syphilis A contagious disease present worldwide, transmitted mainly but not exclusively by sexual contact, caused by the *Treponema pallidum* and resulting in a specific serological reaction (revealed by the Wassermann test).
Cf. sexually transmitted diseases

T

Taboo A prohibition, an unacceptable thing, belief or behaviour according to sacred laws or tribal customs.

Taeniasis Parasitic infection, often symptom-free, of the intestinal tract due to beef tapeworm (*Taenia saginata*), pork tapeworm (*T. solium*) or fish tapeworm (*Diphyllobothrium luum*), acquired mainly through eating insufficiently cooked meat.
Sn: tapeworm infection
also teniasis
Cf. parasitic diseases

Tapeworm Cf. taeniasis

Tar ball Concretion of petroleum following oil slicks. The spilled oil spreads and breaks into smaller patches, which mix with water and emulsify into a sticky substance, under the influence of wind and waves becoming tar balls that can travel great distances, spreading the pollution. Example: the Gulf of Mexico BP oil disaster.
Cf. oil spill

Target The outcome of a plan or action to be attained that should be possible to verify objectively.

Taro A tropical plant, the root of which is used as food, particularly in the Pacific Islands.
Cf. conventional food, staple food

Teaching Eye Surgery Foundation TES is an NGO active in teaching and practising affordable eye surgery mainly in the Indian Ocean area and Mauritius.
Cf. mercy ships.

Tear gas/Tear bomb A variety of gases, including pepper sprays, which are temporarily incapacitating but not lethal, used by police in riot control. Also used by lawless individuals in attacking citizens. Unlike war gases, these gases are usually not prohibited.
Cf. incapacitating agent, riot control

Technical assistance The system of providing assistance, on a bilateral or multilateral basis, through technicians, experts, teachers or equipment, to a developing country.
Sn: technical cooperation (now the preferred term)
Cf. international assistance, bilateral cooperation

Technical cooperation The provision by a technically advanced country, on a bilateral or multilateral basis, of technicians, experts, know-how and equipment, to a country that needs them in order to ensure its social and economic development.

Sn: technical assistance

Cf. development, international assistance, TCDC, technology transfer

Technical cooperation among developing countries/TCDC The promotion of technical cooperation not from developed to developing country, but between developing countries, for the development of both.

Sn: TCDC

Cf. development, technical cooperation, technology transfer

Technological   disaster Man-made disaster due to a sudden or slow mechanical breakdown, technical fault, design error, mistake or involuntary or voluntary human acts that constitute a technological hazard and which cause destruction, death, pollution and environmental damage.

Cf. disaster, man-made disaster, major technological accident, human failure

Technology enabled knowledge translation/TEKT An advanced system using the technical advantages and connectivity of modern information and communication technologies to enable and support evidence-based health knowledge into routine health protection for the overall improvement of health and health delivery – K. Ho.

Cf. telematics, telemedicine

Technology   transfer Transmission from a technologically developed country to one less advanced in economic, industrial or other techniques, of information, knowledge, equipment and training facilities,

with the view to strengthening a particularly weak sector or promoting general development in the receiving country.

Cf. international assistance, technical cooperation, appropriate technology

Tectonic earthquake Cf. plate tectonics, earthquake

Telecommunication Transmission, emission or reception at a distance, of signs, signals, messages, imagery, sounds or any other information by wire, radio, laser, optics, satellite, Internet or other system.

Cf. International Telecommunication Union, social network

Telematics/Telehealth/Telemedicine Also health telematics, telemedicine, telehealth. Telecommunications for health-related activities, services, systems, carried out over a distance by means of information and communication technologies, for the purposes of global health promotion, disease control and health care, as well as education, management and research for health – WHO.

Sn: eHealth

Telematic techniques can also be applied in many other fields.

Telemedicine Cf. telematics/telehealth

Telemetry The measuring of distances, obtained by a stationary receiving station through acoustical, optical and radio-electric procedures.

Telenursing The use of telecommunications and telemedicine facilities for nursing care.

Cf. telematics, telemedicine

Telesurgery The use of telematic technology for on-site computer aided surgery, remote operations and robotic surgery. Also e-Surgery.

Cf. telematics, surgical procedures, essential surgery

Temperature   inversion Sudden increase in the vertical gradient of temperature in the atmosphere.
Cf. atmosphere, stratosphere

Ten-ninety gap/The 10/90 disequilibrium Huge sums, amounting to billions of dollars, are spent on health and health research. However, less than 10% of these are devoted to diseases or conditions that account for 90% of the global diseases or to conditions that account for 90% of the global disease burden, a misallocation that reveals and widens the gap between the healthy and the sick and between the developed and developing countries – WHO.
Cf. burden of disease, technology transfer, orphan diseases

Tephra Ashes and fragments of pyroclastic material ejected by the explosion of volcanic bombs.
Cf. ash, volcano

Terracing Horizontal cuts, benches or embankments made along hillsides to reduce erosion, improve cropping, hold back run-off, improve rain infiltration or other conservation function – OFDA.

Terrestrial longitude Cf. geographic longitude

Territorial asylum Temporary or permanent admission by a State, on its territory, given to a refugee or asylum seeker.
Cf. asylum, diplomatic asylum, refugee

Terrorism Term referring to various kinds of criminal acts of violence, especially against non-combat civilians, such as bombing, setting fire, abducting, poisoning, intimidating, hijacking, killing and other forms of illegal occult actions, with the aim of creating terror, panic or submission among the public, state or individuals. Some forms are bioterrorism, environmental terrorism, political terrorism.
A UN definition is any act by which pain or suffering, whether physical or mental, is intentionally inflicted on a person with such purposes as obtaining from him/her or third person information or a confession, punishing him/her for an act he/she or third person is suspected of having committed or intimidating them.
Cf. arson, hijacking, kleptocracy, piracy, mafia, bioterrorism, booby trap

Tertiary health care The superior level of health-care facilities where highly complicated and specialized conditions that cannot be treated at the general secondary health-care level are referred to for study and treatment.
Cf. primary health care, secondary health care

Tetanus A non-epidemic, highly toxiinfectious, often fatal disease, due to the contamination of wounds or burns or the newborn's umbilicus with *Clostridium tetani* or its spores. Vaccination protects and is included in the WHO programme of immunization.
Cf. Expanded Programme on Immunization

Thalidomide A drug that, given to women during pregnancy, in the 1960s, caused a worldwide pharmaceutical disaster, with thousands of babies born with serious body defects, flippers instead of limbs and other abnormalities. Prior unbiased research is always essential to avoid such disasters.
Cf. technological disaster, bioethics

The Hunger Project An international NGO committed to the elimination of hunger in the world, particularly in the developing countries and in difficult situations. It promotes nutritional studies and agricultural projects and searches for solutions. It is not a relief organization.

Cf. hunger, aridity, drought, famine, Food and Agriculture Organization

Thermal agent disaster Disaster causing severe losses in human lives and material goods as a result of massive heat production. It indicates the relationship between the cause of the event (massive heat production) and its consequences on man and the material environment, as a mathematical expression of the damage caused, i.e. the number of dead and injured and the extent of material damage – Masellis.

Cf. burn disaster, burn, burn centre

Thermograph Thermometer fitted with a device for continuously recording the temperature chronologically on a rotating graph.

Thermonuclear bomb A nuclear weapon in which a part of the explosive power results from fusion reactions, as in the hydrogen bomb.

Sn: hydrogen bomb, fusion bomb

Cf. atomic bomb, fission bomb, nuclear war

Third World Term originally used during the Cold War for the politically non-aligned countries of the world (Group of 77) with allegiance neither to the West nor to the Communist bloc. The term has extended to refer generally to the lower-middle income countries. It is becoming meaningless.

Threatened epidemic A situation in which an epidemic of a specific disease may be reasonably anticipated because of (a) the existence of a susceptible population, or (b) the presence or impending introduction of a disease agent and (c) circumstances, e.g. contaminated water supply, that make such transmission possible – Brès.

Sn: potential epidemic

Cf. epidemic, WHO epidemic alert degrees

Three Mile Island accident A place near Harrisburg, Pennsylvania, USA, site of a nuclear reactor which failed during mechanical handling, on 28 March 1979, causing the most serious nuclear industry accident up to that date, with partial meltdown of fuel rods and some release of radioactive gases. Accident rated as level 5 on the INES scale. Commonly referred to as TMI.

Cf. Chernobyl, Fukushima, nuclear reactor, technological disaster, International Nuclear Event Scale

Threshold A limit below which a reaction does not occur. A level below which danger increases.

In disease statistics, critical threshold denotes reduction of health facilities below which the crude mortality rate increases.

Threshold State A country considered to have a high potential of becoming a nuclear-weapon State either because of its scientific, technical and economic development, e.g. Brazil, or due to its political and military motives, e.g. North Korea. South Africa has voluntarily discontinued its threshold status.

Cf. nuclear war

Thunderstorm A sudden, local, relatively short cloudburst of cumulus with lightning and rumble but usually without a frontal system.

Cf. frontal thunderstorm

Tick-borne typhus One of a group of acute, febrile rickettsial diseases transmitted by ticks, with manifestations similar to typhus.

Cf. rickettsial fever, typhus

Tidal range Sn: amplitude tidal range

Tidal wave Catastrophic wave(s) arriving on the coast accompanied with strong winds and storm surge.

The term is commonly used for the huge waves associated with submarine earthquake and tsunami, but technically, it should be reserved to waves associated with tides, i.e. due to lunar effect.

Cf. tide, storm surge, tsunami

Tide The periodic rise and fall of the earth's oceans and seas due to the attraction by the moon and the sun. The cycle is generally about 12–24 h.

Cf. amplitude tidal range

Tide coefficient Cf. coefficient of tide

Tide forecast Prediction for a particular place, of the height of the tide at a given time or of the heights and times of high and low tides. (Printed in tide tables.)

Sn: tide prediction

Tide land Low coastal land partly under sea water, at least at high tide, and possessing special ecological characteristics.

Sn: tidal wetland

Tide-generating force The resultant of the astral attraction on a particle and of the inertia force of that particle in its movement on the terrestrial orbit.

Cf. force, tidal wave

Tissue engineering The use of bioengineering theories and techniques to design, create, apply materials and devices that replace tissues which have been impaired or have lost function, e.g. artificial skin.

TNT The popular abbreviation for the chemical explosive trinitrotoluene used in conventional weapons. Also used as reference to measure the energy liberated in the explosion of nuclear weapons. Thus, a 1 Mt nuclear bomb has the destructive capacity of one million tons of TNT.

Cf. nuclear bomb, trinitrotoluene

Tobin tax With the aim of introducing more equity and some fairness to less prosperous countries in global monetary mechanisms, a currency transaction tax (CTT) known as the Tobin tax has been proposed – not generally operational to date.

Topography

1. The fixed characteristics and physical features of an area, particularly portraying elevations and landmarks.
2. The geographic science of mapping the positions, elevations, forms, dimensions and other elements of the fixed and permanent features of the surface of the ground at a given time.

Tornado The North American name for a violent whirling wind, generally cyclonic in direction, about 100 m in diameter and extremely destructive in its path. It is measured by the Fujita-Pearson scale.

Sn: twister

Cf. twister, Fujita-Pearson scale.

Torture Any act by which pain and acute physical or mental suffering are intentionally inflicted upon a person in order to obtain a confession or information, to punish for an act committed by him or another suspected person, to intimidate, degrade or exercise pressure, or for any other discriminatory motive, when such pain and suffering are inflicted by a public servant or any other person acting on behalf of an official, with or without the latter's consent – UN Convention Against Torture, 1984. In 2002, the UN adopted the Optional Protocol to the Convention, making it possible to take further measures against torture. Amnesty International, the Association for Prevention of Torture and the Robben Island Guidelines are strong initiatives.

Cf. Geneva Conventions, International Humanitarian Law, United Nations, International Association for Humanitarian Medicine, Robben Island, man-conceived disaster, OPCAT, APT

Totem / Totemism Derived from the Ojibway *Ototomen*, the word means kin or relation, expressing the belief that all individuals have an animal kinship and thus trotemic representation in the spiritual world; a non-religious clan or personal concept of animal ties with the supernmatural, without the need of a shaman , medium or priestly intermediary. In certain areas, as among the First Nations of North-West America, privileged initiates can act as medicine-men. – Kwe Kwala Gila

Cf. shamanism, traditional medicine, aborigine

Toxic chemical The Chemical Weapons Convention defines a "toxic chemical" as any chemical which through its chemical action on life processes can cause death, temporary incapacitation or permanent harm to humans and animals. This includes all such chemicals regardless of their origin or of their method of production and regardless of whether they are produced in facilities, in munitions or elsewhere – CWC.

Cf. chemical weapons, Chemical Weapons Convention, biological weapons, chemical warfare

Toxicological disaster Serious environmental pollution and illness caused by the massive accidental escape of toxic substances into the air, soil or water and to man, animals or plants.

Cf. toxic chemical, dioxin, man-made disaster, Seveso, Bhopal, technological disaster, major accident hazard

Toxicology The science of poisons, harmful chemical substances, organic toxins and of their detection, effect, elimination and antidotes.

Cf. toxicological disaster.

Toxin Substance secreted by certain living organisms, capable of causing harmful (toxic) effects in the receiving organism.

Trace elements Chemical and mineral elements, usually beneficial, that exist in minimal traces (oligo-quantities) in various media, e.g. the body, in foods, in the air, in soil.

Sn: oligo-elements

Trachoma A contagious viral eye disease (keratoconjunctivitis), endemic in many countries where it is a major cause of blindness. A neglected tropical disease.

Trade wind Regular winds that blow throughout the year between the tropical high pressures and the equatorial low pressures.

Cf. atmospheric pressure

Traditional birth attendant A person who assists the mother at childbirth and who initially acquires her skill of delivering babies by herself or by working with other traditional birth attendants – WHO.

(In contrast to midwife who requires a formal medical education.)

Traditional medicine Local folk medicine, native indigenous healing. "…It is part of the tradition of each country and employs practices that are handed down from generation to generation of healers. Its acceptance by people receiving care is also inherited from generation to generation" – WHO/SEARO.

Transboundary pollution Pollution and pollutants that have been produced in one country and that have passed international boundaries through water or air to other countries, causing pollution. The effects can be mitigated only through international agreements as the damage is caused outside the boundaries of the victim's country.
Sn: transfrontier pollution
Cf. acid rain, Chernobyl, ozone depletion, global health

Transform fault Sn: sliding fault

Transit centre A centre which houses refugees (or other disaster victims) awaiting the completion of formalities for departure.

Transmission (of disease) The passage of a disease – commonly an infectious disease, less commonly a hereditary condition – from one individual to another.
Sn: disease transmission
Cf. communicable disease, infectious disease, carrier

Transparency International/TI An NGO founded in 1993 that seeks out and publicizes corruption in political, international and corporate bodies with the view to promoting transparency and fairness in development. Publishes the annual "Corporate Perceptions Index" which compares and ranks corruption worldwide.
Cf. transparent

Transparent Vision: Easily seen through; bright.
Social: Person or statement without affectation, lie or disguise.
Organization/government: Political, governmental or corporate activity whose record is clear, accountable, not corrupt.
Cf. Transparency International, glasnost

Transuranium elements Elements, such as plutonium, neptunium, that occur above uranium in the periodic table, generated in nuclear power reactors. They also disperse dangerously following atom bomb tests.
Cf. uranium, plutonium, nuclear reactor

Trauma/Trauma score Bodily injury due to any cause, any extent and any gravity. The trauma score is a numerical grading system for estimating the severity of injury, each parameter receiving a number (high for normal and low for impaired function). The severity of injury is estimated as the sum total of the numbers, the lowest score being 1 and the highest 16.
Cf. Glasgow coma scale, survival chain

Trauma and injury severity score/ TRISS A physiological and anatomical formula to evaluate the likelihood of survival following severe injuries, marking the probability from 0 to 100%.
Cf. trauma injury classification, Glasgow trauma scale

Trauma, injury classification The ITACCS classification of injuries related to trauma defines the following:
Major injury: Injury severity score >15, comprising at least one severe life-threatening regional injury. OR at least two severe non-life-threatening regional injuries. OR at least two severe non-life-threatening injuries plus at least two injuries of moderate severity.
Multiple trauma/Polytrauma: Injury to one body cavity such as head, thorax, abdomen, plus two long-bone and/or pelvic fractures. OR, plus injury to two body cavities.
Cf. trauma score, ITACCS

Treaty An international contract in writing between two or more States, negotiated, signed, ratified and binding to the States parties. Some terms used interchangeably for the same are covenant, pact, convention, agreement, protocol, international treaty.

Trend analysis A tool in decision-making and quality control that takes one criterion from an operation category and compares it against another criterion over time. The more criteria compared to one another, the more sensitive, reliable and specific will the analysis be. Example: food distribution vs. crude mortality rate analyzed over time – Burkle.

Trial A Swiss association of lawyers and of impunity victims, active in tracking down and denouncing impunity. It aims at putting the law at the service of victims of international crime, such as genocide, war crimes, torture or forced disappearances.

Cf. impunity, war crimes, genocide, torture, disappearance

Triage Selection and categorization of the victims of a disaster with the view to appropriate treatment according to the degree or severity of illness or injury and the availability of medical and transport facilities.

Trinitrotoluene/TNT The chemical name for the explosive TNT, the main substance in conventional weapons. Also used for measuring the energy liberated in the explosion of a nuclear weapon. Thus, a 1 Mt nuclear bomb has the destructive capacity of one million tons of TNT.

Cf. TNT

Tropical air Mass of air which has stayed over tropical latitudes for several days and which, accordingly, has become relatively warm.

Cf. tropical zones

Tropical climate The prevailing climate in the subtropical and tropical zones, characterized by a well-marked dry season (in the months when it is winter in the northern hemisphere) and an equally distinct rainy season (during the summer in the northern hemisphere).

Cf. climate, dry season, rainy season

Tropical cyclone A strong meteorological depression, generated in the tropics and giving rise to extremely violent winds. The term tropical cyclone covers typhoon, hurricane and cyclone. Seasonal cause of disaster. Wind force Beaufort 12, over 58 knots.

In the northern hemisphere, the cyclonic winds spin counterclockwise around a warm centre core, the eye, while in the southern hemisphere, they rotate clockwise.

Cf. cyclone, hurricane, typhoon

Tropical depression Tropical perturbance with maximum winds below 34 knots.

Cf. depression, tropical storm, wind

Tropical Health and Education Trust/ THET An organization that promotes and conducts training programmes for frontier health-care and essential surgical workers, particularly in Egypt, tropical and developing countries.

Cf. essential surgery

Tropical storm

1. Any tropical cyclonic disturbance.
2. Tropical cyclone with maximum winds between 34 and 64 knots.

Cf. cyclone, tropical cyclone, tropical depression

Tropical zones Countries which are continually warm, situated between the tropical latitudes, where the seasonal differentiation is in function of the rainfall, expressed as a dry season (corresponding to winter in the northern hemisphere) and a humid season.

Cf. rainfall, rainy season, dry season, season

Troposphere The region of the atmosphere immediately above the earth's surface in which the temperature falls with increasing altitude.

Truth and Reconciliation Commission: TRC/SA Following the demise of the apartheid regime in South Africa in1994, the new Constitution and Bill of Rights introduced the bold pioneering concept of a national Truth and Reconciliation Commission as part of the country's peaceful transformation and establishment of democracy. It granted "amnesty in respect of acts, omissions and offences associated with political objectives and committed in the course of conflicts of the past". Cf. ICTR. Compare with the UN-created International Criminal Tribunal for Rwanda

Trypanosomiasis Sn: sleeping sickness

Tsunami Huge ocean waves generated by an underwater upheaval such as submarine earthquake or volcanic eruption. The waves move out fast in all directions over hundreds of miles, causing great destruction. The worst recent tsunami occurred on 26 December 2004, off Sumatra, Indonesia, spreading as far west as the African coast, causing over 250,000 deaths. In 2011, the concurrent tsunami-earthquake-nuclear meltdown at Fukushima-Daiichi, Japan, was the worst compound disaster. Cf. seismic sea wave, tidal wave, compound disaster

Tuberculosis/TB/Tb Infectious and contagious disease, with particular localization in the lungs, caused by the *Mycobacterium tuberculosis.* BCG vaccination is important, but the disease is still endemic in many regions and a real hazard in crowded unsanitary

conditions following disaster. One of the six diseases in the WHO immunization programme. In recent years, it has been spreading in a virulent form with, currently, new attack strategies. Commonly used abbreviation: TB.

Active TB: Positive presence of the signs, symptoms and findings of the disease.

– Infectious TB: Active TB with the infection transmissible to others.

– Latent TB: Bacteriology and laboratory tests positive but no clinical evidence of the disease.

– Multi-drug resistant TB: TB strains resistant to at least isoniazid and rifampicin (MDR-TB). Cf. Expanded Programme on Immunization, The Global Fund

Twister Sn: tornado

Typhoid fever A serious enteric infectious disease, transmitted by patients, carriers, water or food, such as contaminated shellfish. It is characterized by fever, slow pulse, skin eruption, abdominal signs, enlarged spleen and prostration. Many enteric diseases are labelled typhoid fever, but the latter only is caused by *Salmonella typhi.*
It is a popular belief that typhoid frequently follows floods and other disasters; it is in fact unusual, and mass vaccination is not recommended. Personal hygienic practices constitute the best prevention. (Do not confuse typhoid with typhus.) Cf. diarrhoeal diseases, enteric diseases, carrier, oral rehydration, salmonellosis

Typhoon A Chinese term, now universally adopted, for tropical cyclone in the Western Pacific, same as "hurricane" in the Atlantic and "cyclone" in South East Asia. Winds force 12 Beaufort, over 58 knots. Cf. cyclone, hurricane, tropical cyclone

Typhoon   warning Meteorological message to warn of the existence or expected arrival of a typhoon, often coupled with advice on protective measures.

Cf. cyclone, hurricane, typhoon, weather forecast

Typhus One of the serious rickettsial fevers, the classically notorious epidemic typhus, transmitted by lice. Immunization and louse control are highly effective. (Not to be confused with typhoid.)

Cf. rickettsial fever, tick-borne typhus, typhus exanthematicus

Typhus exanthematicus Cf. rickettsial fever, typhus

Tziganes Groups of populations believed to have originated in India and since the sixteenth century spread across Europe, living mostly in a nomadic manner, without fixed residence, defined state or boundaries. Much discriminated against, they deserve all human rights. The Schengen accords on free movement in Europe apply to them also. Without clear distinction, they are also variously known as Gypsies, Roma, Sinti, travellers.

Cf. nomad, racism, discrimination, human rights

U

Unaccompanied minor A child under 15 years of age who has been separated from both parents following a disaster, exodus or refugee displacement and for whose care no person can be found who by law or custom has primary responsibility. Humanitarian organizations usually take care of unaccompanied minors/children pending family reunion. (It is the usual practice of UNHCR to allow unaccompanied children over 15 to take decisions concerning durable solutions for themselves).

Sn: unaccompanied child

Cf. Refugee, Rädda Barnen, child

UNAIDS Acronym for Joint United Nations Programme on HIV/AIDS, the principal worldwide programme on all aspects of financing, monitoring, research, evaluation and treatment of this pandemic. (It has affinities to but should not be confused with UNITAID.)

Undernutrition

1. Inadequate intake of food, hence of energy, over a period of time.
2. Pathological state arising from inadequate intake of food and hence of calories, over a considerable period, manifest by reduced body weight.

Cf. energy requirements, malnutrition, famine

UN hazard classification 9 Classes: (1) explosive, mass explosion hazard, very insensitive substances; (2) flammable gases, non-flammable non-toxic gases, toxic gases; (3) flammable liquids; (4) flammable solids, spontaneously combustible substances, substances dangerous when wet; (5) oxidizing substances other than organic peroxides, organic peroxides; (6) poisonous (toxic) substances, infectious substances; (7) radioactive substances; (8) corrosive substances and (9) other dangerous substances – IPCS.

Cf. chemical accident, major accident hazard, Bhopal, Seveso, environmental pollution, IPCS, Basel Convention, hazardous material

United Nations/UN The supreme intergovernmental world body established in 1945 with the purposes of (1) maintaining international peace and security, (2) developing friendly relations among nations, (3) solving international problems through international cooperation and (4) harmonizing the actions of all nations for these common ends. The UN acts through various mechanisms, such as specialized agencies, e.g. WHO; Councils, e.g. for Human Rights at UNHCHR; High Commission Offices, e.g. UNHCR for Refugees; Committees, e.g. on Atomic Radiation, Funds, e.g. UNICEF; major programmes, e.g. UNDP; peacekeeping forces, e.g. UNIFIL; institutes, e.g. UNITAR

OCHA is responsible for the direction and coordination of the UN response and capability in natural and other disasters. The following UN bodies are involved in disaster assistance:

Cf. UN Office for the Coordination of Humanitarian Affairs (OCHA); Food and Agriculture Organization (FAO); International Atomic Energy Agency (IAEA); High Commissioner for Human Rights (HCHR); International Telecommunication Union (ITU); United Nations Children's Fund (UNICEF); United Nations Development Programme (UNDP); United Nations Educational, Scientific and Cultural Organization (UNESCO); United Nations Environment Programme (UNEP); United Nations High Commissioner for Refugees (UNHCR); United Nations Relief and Works Agency for Palestine Refugees (UNRWA); World Food Programme (WFP); World Health Organization (WHO); World Meteorological Organization (WMO). (See these organizations separately.) The UN also maintains non-governmental relations (NGLS/NGO).

United Nations Headquarters/Secretariat The main seat of the United Nations, situated in New York. Houses the General Assembly building, the Executive Office of the Secretary-General and the main political bodies of the UN that establish the general policies and provide overall guidance to the organization. There are three other main UN offices in Geneva, Vienna and Nairobi.

United Nations Office at Geneva/UNOG Second largest UN establishment, housing mainly the centres for conferences, diplomacy, disarmament, human rights, refugees, disasters, specialized agencies for health, telecommunications, labour, intellectual property, meteorology. Inter alia, seat of the Office of the High Commissioner for Human Rights and of the Office for the Coordination of Humanitarian Affairs.

Cf. OHCHR, OHCR, OCHA

United Nations Office at Nairobi/UNON Headquarters for activities in the fields of environment and human settlements. Seat of UNEP.

United Nations Office at Vienna/UNOV Headquarters for activities in the fields of nuclear energy, drug control, crime prevention, international trade law. Seat of the International Atomic Energy Agency.

United Nations Office for the Coordination of Humanitarian Affairs/OCHA Better known by its acronym OCHA, principal Office under the direction of the UN Emergency Relief Coordinator, for the organization and operation of the UN capability for assessing, responding to and managing natural and other disasters. It includes ISDR, the International Strategy for Disaster Reduction. Operates in coordination with other UN, NGO and expert bodies, including WHO, FAO, HCR, UNICEF, ITU, UNEP, WFP, WMO, UNDP.

Sn: OCHA, previously UNDRO

Cf. see these organizations separately, ISDR

UNFCCC Cf. United Nations Framework Convention on Climate Change, global warming, glasshouse effect, climate change

United Nations Children's Fund/ UNICEF Better known by its acronym UNICEF, principal organization that acts to protect children's rights; ensures that children get the best possible start in life and grow harmoniously. Collaborates with WHO in primary health care. Protects children's rights in disasters.

Sn: UNICEF

Cf. rights of the child, primary health care

United Nations Civilian Police/ UNCIVPOL Civilian police, mainly UN civilian police, are being increasingly employed in post-conflict situations and reconstruction stabilization efforts. To the traditional work of monitoring, observing and reporting are now added such tasks as reforming and restructuring of local forces, training, advice and sometimes law enforcement. But they do not carry out executive policing.

Cf. democratic control of armed forces

UNICEF Acronym for United Nations Children's Fund. Name most commonly used instead of the longer title.

Unilateralism The position of one State, acting singly in the international arena and in international affairs, on its own initiative without consideration of the position or agreement of others. The opposite is bilateralism and multilateralism.

United Nations Democracy Fund/ UNDEF A voluntary fund with the purpose of investing in democratization processes and thus encouraging the progress of nations towards the ideals and practice of democracy.

Cf. democracy, development

United Nations Department of Peacekeeping Operations/DPKO Key activity in the UN for mounting and operating peacekeeping actions and humanitarian ceasefire orders. Also serves as the focal point for mine action.

Cf. humanitarian, antipersonnel mines

United Nations Development Programme/UNDP The principal UN programme for multilateral technical and pre-investment cooperation for development. The funding source for most of the technical assistance provided by the UN. Represents OCHA in disaster situations.

Cf. development, technical assistance, Millennium Development Goals

United Nations Economic and Social Commission for Asia and the Pacific/ESCAP UN Commission to facilitate regional economic development in the Asia-Pacific region, to alleviate poverty; strengthen the environment, transport, communications; help least developed countries and maintain good relations among the region's nations.

Similar Economic and Social Commissions apply also to Africa (UNECA), Europe (UNECE), Latin

America and the Caribbean (ECLAC) and Western Asia (ESCWA).

United Nations Educational, Scientific and Cultural Organization/ UNESCO Better known by its acronym UNESCO, the lead organization for education, cultural development and cultural heritage, press freedom, human sciences, natural sciences, environmental research. Is the depository of information on earthquakes and has a programme on the protection of the lithosphere.
Cf. earthquake, culture

UNESCO Acronym and the usual term used for United Nations Educational, Scientific and Cultural Organization.

United Nations Environment Programme/UNEP Special programme of the UN to promote a harmonious interrelationship between environment and development, by wise and technically sound utilization of resources and by reducing the degradation and pollution of the environment. Acts in natural environment catastrophes (earthquake, drought, deforestation) and man-made disasters (chemical explosion, oil spill, pollution).
Sn: UNEP
Cf. deforestation, environment, United Nations

United Nations Framework Convention on Climate Change/ UNFCCC Scientific and organizational efforts to stabilize greenhouse gas concentration, to ensure that food production and sea levels are not threatened and to enable the continuity of sustainable development.
Cf. greenhouse effect, Kyoto protocol, climate change

United Nations High Commissioner for Human Rights/ UNHCHR UNHCHR has a wide mandate covering all aspects of human rights as enshrined in the Universal Declaration of Human Rights. Inter alia, it promotes the right to development, recognition of social, economic and cultural rights, gender equality, and the rights of the child and helps states implement human rights plans and actions. Through its Council on Human Rights, it oversees and evaluates a state's obligations in implementing human rights and calls for correction of breaches of human rights.
Sn: UNHCHR, also OHCHR, HCHR
Cf. Universal Declaration of Human Rights, UN Human Rights Council

United Nations Human Rights Council/HRC Created in March 2006 as successor to the Human Rights Commission, this is a permanent intergovernmental body of 47 States, responsible for the examination, promotion and protection of human rights around the globe, within the Office of the High Commissioner for Human Rights.
Cf. United Nations High Commissioner for Human Rights

United Nations Institute for Disarmament Research/UNIDIR In cooperation with the UN Department of Disarmament Affairs, UNIDIR provides member states with objective research on all aspects of disarmament and on all forms of human security.

United Nations Non-Governmental Liaison Service UN/NGLS An inter-agency programme of the UN mandated to promote and develop constructive relations between the United Nations and civil society non-governmental organizations (NGLS).

Cf. civil society, NGOs, voluntary organizations

United Nations Office on Drugs and Crime/UNODC Addresses the worldwide issues of narcotics trafficking, drug control, crime prevention and international terrorism in all forms. It consists of the UN Drug Control Programme and the Centre for International Crime Prevention at Vienna.

Cf. drug trafficking, Palermo protocol, Farc, terrorism

United Nations Sudano-Sahelian Office/UNSO Integrates dry land problems into national development programmes. Is concerned with dry lands and poverty, drought preparedness and mitigation, land tenure, knowledge in and management of desertification

United Nations Millennium Declaration To encourage improvements and modernization of the 60-year-old United Nations and to accelerate development for all peoples in the coming century, the General Assembly in 2000 adopted the Millennium Declaration, with ambitious programmes to usher in the twenty-first century. Of these, the principal initiative that continues is the significant programme of Millennium Development Goals, MDGs, with eight specific objectives for 2000–2015.

Cf. Millennium Development Goals, United Nations, AIFOMD, development

United Nations Population Fund/ UNFPA The world's largest international source of financing for reproductive health programmes, population studies and related disease and social issues. A key goal is to reduce maternal mortality by 75% by 2015.

United Nations Relief and Works Agency for Palestine Refugees in the Near East Full official designation for UNRWA.

UNRWA is the popular acronymic term used for the agency.

United Nations Scientific Committee on the Effects of Atomic Radiation/ UNSCEAR Set up in 1955, official scientific body to evaluate doses, effects, risks and remote dangers of radiation from any source on a worldwide basis.

Sn: UNSCEAR

Cf. radiation, atomic war, Hiroshima, Fukushima, GLAWARS

UNISDR Cf. International Strategy for Disaster Reduction, Office for the Coordination of Humanitarian Affairs, OCHA

UNITAID/WHO Launched at the World Health Organization, it is essentially an international drug purchasing facility to acquire affordable medicines and diagnostics mainly to combat HIV/AIDS, malaria and tuberculosis. An imaginative aspect is that it is financed primarily through the proceeds of a tax levied on airline tickets, which ensures a fair and steady flow of funds.

United Nations University/ UNU Academic centre in Tokyo for advanced training and knowledge in all aspects of the UN's concerns, in particular peace and governance and sustainable development. Publishes a wide array of studies and books in these fields.

Cf. UNU World Institute for Development Economics Research

UNU World Institute for Development Economics Research/UNU-WIDER The economics research arm of the United Nations University, with particular interest in poverty and inequality, refugees, migration, social development, globalization, finance and growth.

Cf. United Nations University, Millennium Development Goals

United Nations Watch Believing in the beneficial mission of the United Nations, this non-profit NGO undertakes the task of monitoring and watching over the performance of the UN and its adherence to the UN Charter and any eventual shortcomings.

Cf. United Nations, NGO

Universal Declaration of Human Rights/UDHR Universal declaration, proclaimed on 10 December 1948, by the United Nations General Assembly, guaranteeing every citizen certain inalienable rights, through the 30 separate articles, as follows:

1. The right to equality
2. Freedom from discrimination
3. The right to life, liberty and personal security
4. Freedom from slavery
5. Freedom from torture or degrading treatment
6. The right to recognition as a person before the law
7. The right to equality before the law
8. The right to fairness by a competent tribunal
9. Freedom from arbitrary arrest or exile
10. The right to a fair and public hearing
11. The right to be considered innocent until proven guilty
12. Freedom from interference with privacy, family, home or correspondence
13. The right to free movement in and out of any country
14. The right to asylum in other countries from persecution
15. The right to a nationality and freedom to change it
16. The right to marriage and family
17. The right to own property
18. Freedom of belief and religion
19. Freedom of opinion and information
20. The right of peaceful assembly and association
21. The right to participate in government and free elections
22. The right to social security
23. The right to a desiderable work and to join trade unions
24. The right to rest and leisure
25. The right to an adequate standard of living
26. The right to education
27. The right to participate in the cultural life of a community
28. The right to social order assuring human rights
29. The right to community duties that are essential to free and full development
30. Freedom from state or personal interference in the above rights

Universal health coverage Equitable provision of and access to health care for all citizens, at all ages and for all health conditions and services, ensuring social health protection for all.

Cf. national health service, Health for All, access to health

Universality of human rights The doctrine that all human rights are held unconditionally by all humans without distinction. (A contrary view is held by a minority doctrine of cultural relativism.) But human rights are universal, indivisible and apply to all persons of all cultures and creeds.

Cf. Universal Declaration of Human Rights, cultural relativism

Universal suffrage The political human right of every adult citizen to vote for or against a principal institution or an agent of the State. Certain institutions oppose this right on the basis of cultural relativism.

Cf. cultural relativism, universality of human rights, empower

Universal Time Coordinated/ UTC The coordinated time recorded by an official uniformly running clock, the measure of Greenwich mean time corrected for seasonal variations in the earth's rotation.

Sn: UTC

Cf. Greenwich mean time, GMT

Universitas-21/U-21 U-21. A consortium of initially 21 (now more) universities representing academics, scientists, sociologists, doctors, students and other intellectuals concerned with international higher education, high social standards, the UN, development and academic freedom.

Cf. ACUNS

Unnecessary suffering According to International Humanitarian Law, it refers to inflicting physical, mental or psychological suffering which exceeds that needed to neutralize an enemy irrespective of the weapon used.

Cf. law of war

UNRWA Modified acronym and usual term for United Nations Relief and Works Agency for Palestine Refugees, organization that since 1950 has been assisting and protecting Palestine refugees – who are not included in UNHCR's mandate.

Cf. refugee, UNHCR, United Nations

UNSCEAR Sn: United Nations Scientific Committee on the Effects of Atomic Radiation

Cf. refugee, nuclear reactor, atom bomb

Upper-middle income country The World Bank (2008) categorizes countries according to gross national income (GNI, previously GNP) per capita: upper-middle income country: US\$3,856–1,1905.

Cf. emerging countries, developed countries, high-income countries, country income categories, least developed countries

Uranium/U235/U308 A mineral element that exists in the soil as 0.7% U235, symbol U, atomic number 92. This is the only naturally occurring fissile isotope and, with due processing, is used for military and civilian nuclear reactors. Extracted from the soil, it is purified by removal of the gangue. The concentrate thus obtained is U308, a powder also known as "yellow cake". To utilize this for civilian or military purposes, it is further transformed into uranium fluoride (UF6). For use in reactors, this needs further "enrichment" to go much higher than 0.7%. The process is physical, utilizing a great number of successively powerful centrifuges. For civilian use, 5% of U235 is needed. For military use (atom bomb), more than 90% is required. This process is highly controlled by the UN International Atomic Energy Agency. The atom bomb dropped on Hiroshima was of the uranium type.

Cf. atom bomb, Hiroshima, plutonium, caesium, posturanium elements, nuclear reactor, IAEA Smb: U

Uranium enrichment Enhancing uranium for military purposes. Process highly controlled by Treaty and by the IAEA.

Cf. uranium

Urbanization Transformation of rural land to urban use, under the influence of economic, demographic and spatial pressures of an urban centre, with consequent problems.
Cf. conurbation

Utilities failure Sudden breakdown of public utilities, including electricity, telephone, Internet, water supplies, pipelines, refrigeration systems, etc., due mainly to power failure or other malfunction, causing a serious emergency. In a disaster, such failures are a part of the damage and complicate the situation further.

Utstein standards Named after a centre of study, research, contemplation and conference in Norway, where standardization templates and quality control systems are formulated and proposed, particularly concerning the quality of management in various emergencies. Example: the Task Force on Quality Control in Disasters, initiated by the Nordic Society for Disaster Medicine and the World Association for Disaster and Emergency Medicine.
Cf. WADEM, disaster management, damage probability formula

V

Vaccination Method of preventing certain infectious diseases by conferring active immunity in a person through the introduction – by injection/ingestion/application – of certain preparations called vaccines, which reinforce the resistance of the body.
Sn: immunization
Cf. infection, vaccine

Vaccine Antigenic preparation that has the property of causing the formation of protective antibodies in the receiver, used for the prevention of certain microbial, viral or parasitic diseases by vaccination.
Cf. immunization, vaccination

Varicella Chickenpox. Highly contagious viral infection, mainly among children.

VD Popular abbreviation for venereal disease. Sexually transmitted disease.
Sn: venereal disease

Vector Medicine: Animal or insect that acts as intermediate host or carrier, transmitting disease from one to another, especially to humans.
Cf. carrier, infection, transmission
Ballistics: A missile that carries a military nuclear device.

Vegetation fire(s) Term covering fires of all types of vegetation, such as forest, grassland brush, woodland, wildland or agricultural.
Cf. forest/vegetation fires

Vehicle In medicine, an object, e.g. an infected handkerchief, an animal, e.g. a dog, or a pathogen, e.g. a virus, that acts as a medium of transmission of disease.
Cf. vector

Venereal disease Disease transmitted by the genital tract. The classically mentioned are syphilis and gonorrhoea, but there are many others, now named under sexually transmitted diseases, including HIV/AIDS.
Sn: VD
Cf. sexually transmitted diseases

Verruga (peruana) Sn: bartonellosis

Vienna Convention, 1969 According to jus cogens, customary norms become acceptable as law.
Cf. jus cogens

Vienna Declaration,1993 The Vienna Declaration and Programme of Action, adopted in 1993, fights against impunity, to provide a firm

base for the rule of law, to punish all those responsible for violations of such acts as torture. Gives power to the Human Rights Council to despatch Commissions of Inquiry when governments are unwilling to investigate human rights violations.
Cf. impunity, Universal Declaration of Human Rights

Violence The intentional use of physical force or power, threatened or actual, against oneself, or another person or against a group or community that either results in or has a high likelihood of resulting in injury, death, psychological harm, maldevelopment or deprivation – WHO.

Violence against women Any act of gender-based violence that results in, or is likely to result in, physical, sexual or psychological harm or suffering to women, including threats of such acts, coercion or arbitrary deprivation of liberty, whether occurring in public or private life – UN.
Cf. female genital mutilation, violence

Violent conflict risk factors Factors that constitute risks of violence among states include, inter alia: lack of democratic process, unequal access to power, social inequality, monopoly of or unequal access to resources, poverty, uncontrolled rapid demographic changes.
Cf. conflict, violence, democracy

Virucide Chemical compound used to destroy viruses.
Cf. pesticide

Virulence The ability of a pathological organism to produce a disease of any degree of seriousness.

Virus Bacteriology: Self-reproducing infectious agent smaller than bacteria, containing only one type of nucleic acid and multiplying only in cells and responsible for a wide range of diseases and often of epidemics.
Cf. epidemic, human immunodeficiency virus, avian influenza, porcine influenza
Information technology: Electronic bug illegally introduced by hackers into a computer system with the view to disrupting the communication.
Cf. cyberwar, hacker

Viral hepatitis (A, B, C) Infection of the liver, due to a virus, probably of three types: type A (previously known as acute infectious hepatitis), type B (usually called serum or post-transfusion hepatitis) and type C (that can be chronic).
Type A is spread mainly by faecal-oral contact and contaminated water or food. It is a real risk in congested, insalubrious areas following disaster. Type B is mainly transmitted through blood transfusions. It has become a major problem among drug addicts through the repeated use of infected needles. Type C predisposes to cancer.

Virgin population A population that has to date not been exposed to a particular infectious organism.

Visceral leishmaniasis A tropical and subtropical parasitic disease transmitted by sandflies.
Sn: kala azar
Cf. leishmaniasis

Vitamin A deficiency Nutritional deficiency in vitamin A or retinol. The leading cause of blindness in infants and xerophthalmia (night blindness).
Sn: hypovitaminosis A

Vitamin B$_1$ deficiency Sn: beriberi, hypovitaminosis B$_1$

Vitamin B$_2$ deficiency A nutritional deficiency due to lack of vitamin B$_2$ (riboflavin) and characterized by tongue and lip lesions.
Sn: ariboflavinosis, hypovitaminosis B$_2$

Vitamin C deficiency Sn: hypovitaminosis C, scurvy

Vitamin D deficiency Sn: hypovitaminosis D, rickets

Vitamin PP deficiency Sn: hypovitaminosis PP, pellagra

Vitamin deficiency Lack of vitamin intake, without specifying the particular vitamin deficiency. There is no deficiency in all vitamins, specific deficiencies lead to specific diseases.
Sn: hypovitaminosis
Cf. beriberi, pellagra, rickets, scurvy, vitamin A deficiency, vitamin B$_1$ deficiency, vitamin B$_2$ deficiency, vitamin C deficiency, vitamin D deficiency

Volcanic eruption The sudden explosive ejection of superheated matter – lava, cinders, ashes, gases and dust – from a volcanic crater or vent.
Cf. volcano

Volcanic risk map The approaches to active volcanoes are divided into three zones according to the degree of risk: exclusion zone: no admittance except for scientific monitoring and national security matters; central zone: residential area only, all residents on heightened state of alert. All residents to have hard hats and masks and to be able to exit within 24 h; impact zone: area with significantly lower risk, suitable for residential and commercial occupation – IDNDR.
Cf. volcanic eruption, risk map, zoning

Volcano A conical mountain with an opening on the earth's crust through which magma of molten rock or gases or both erupt to the surface.
Cf. ash, magma, solfatara, stratovolcano, tephra

Voluntarism A personal or group expression of altruism, providing free assistance and services to persons or people in need.
Cf. altruism, voluntary agency, philanthropy

Voluntary agency Non-profit, non-governmental, private association, maintained and supported by voluntary contributions. Among its activities, assistance in emergencies and disasters is notable. ICVA, the International Council of Voluntary Agencies, represents their federation.
Sn: VOLAG, voluntary organization
Cf. international assistance, altruism

Voluntary organization Sn: voluntary agency.
Cf. non-governmental organization, NGO

Voluntary repatriation The freely consented return of a refugee to his country with the view to his reestablishment there.
Cf. principle of non-refoulement, refugee, repatriation

Vortex The "eye" or centre of the spiral clouds of a cyclone, hurricane or typhoon.

Vulnerable Susceptible to injury, illness, damage or loss. Weak.
Cf. susceptible case, vulnerability

Vulnerability Degree or potential loss (from 0 to 100%) resulting from a possibly harmful phenomenon that causes victims and material damage – After UN-OCHA.
The susceptibility of a person, population, structure or environment to varying degrees of injury or damage,

depending on the assaulting force and the recipient's condition.

In disaster response: A significant weakness in safety or security due to failure in design, structure, maintenance, operation, assessment or age. Cf. susceptible case, vulnerable, elements at risk, hazard

Vulnerability study Study and investigation of all the risks and the hazards susceptible to cause a disaster.

Cf. disaster, hazard, prevention, risk indicator

Vulnerable group A section of the population, especially infants, pregnant and lactating mothers, the elderly, the homeless, who are particularly prone to sickness and nutritional deficiencies. They are likely to suffer most in a disaster.

Vulnerable person Individual who is at risk.

Cf. vulnerable, susceptible case, vulnerable group, risk

Vulnerology From the Latin *vulnus* = wound, injury, damage. A new term for all aspects of study, prevention, treatment and recovery of wounds. – Costagliola Vulnerable is derived from the same root.

Cf. vulnerability, injury, trauma, casualty, violence

W

WADEM/Utstein damage formula Cf. damage probability formula

War A state of declared hostilities, use of force and armed conflict between two or more nations internationally or between parts of one nation, factions or tribes internally. International Humanitarian Law (laws of war), the Geneva Conventions (1947) and the Hague Rules (1907) apply, but in recent years, these rules of conduct have been increasingly breached. War is the worst man-made disaster.

Cf. International Humanitarian Law, International Red Cross, complex disaster, non-violence

War crimes During hostilities, crimes committed in breach of established customs and principles of international law or the laws of war. They include (a) grave breaches of the four Geneva Conventions and their Additional Protocols, such as wilful killing, unnecessarily excessive destruction; (b) other serious violations of the laws and customs applicable to international armed conflicts, such as targeting civilians, pillaging; (c) violations of laws concerning armed conflicts of not an international character, such as cruelty against those not taking part in the conflicts and (d) other serious violations of laws in non-international conflicts, such as attacks on peaceful buildings. War crimes are considered as crimes against humanity and come under the jurisdiction of the International Criminal Court. Cf. crimes against humanity, Geneva Conventions, International Committee of the Red Cross, International Humanitarian Law, man-conceived disaster. International Court of Justice, International Criminal Court

War Crimes Tribunal Cf. International Criminal Court, International Court of Justice, war crimes

War/Law of Sn: International Humanitarian Law

Cf. war, Geneva Conventions

War Trauma Foundation/ WTF Organization that studies and assists in effects of trauma due to war and other disasters. With WHO has produced a guide to strengthen

humanitarian relief especially in psychological first aid.
Cf. post-traumatic stress

War wounded
1. In the strict sense, regular member of the armed forces wounded in an armed conflict in the course of military operations.
2. In a wider sense, any person wounded during an armed conflict in the course of military operations.
3. Handicapped war veteran.
   Cf. armed conflict, Geneva Conventions

Warehouse In transport and shipping, represents a shed or storehouse where cargo is kept pending dispatch or retrieval. Bonded warehouse is an official warehouse under customs control where transit cargo is kept or where cargo is stored pending customs clearance.

Warning Cf. early warning system, alert

Washout Sn: rainout
Cf. scavenging, nuclear explosion

Wastage Misuse of the forces, resources, material, human capabilities and financial means

Waste water Water rendered unsafe and polluted in the course of its domestic or industrial use, comprising household (kitchen, laundry), drainage (lavatories) and residual (industrial) effluents.
Cf. sanitary engineering.

Wasting Depletion of the essential biological, cellular constituents of the body, reflects in the loss of fat and muscle tissue, resulting from prolonged food deprivation and often associated with infections or other diseases.
Sn: emaciation

Water Water is essential to life, for drinking, cooking, personal care and domestic hygiene. Its availability in sufficient quantities and cleanliness is critical in disaster situations, refugee camps and poor environments.
Sn: H_2O

In disaster and refugee situations, the average basic requirement for water is 20 l per person per day.
Cf. water needs

Water harnessing The process of capturing and channelling the water of a spring, lake or river into a network for utilization.
Sn: river basin

Water needs The absolute physiological requirement per person is 1–1.5 l per day. A minimum of 3–5 l daily are necessary for survival in disaster and difficult situations. The average needs are 20 l.
Cf. water, essential bodily needs

Water purification Cf. chlorine, bleaching powder

Waterboarding One barbaric form, among many, of inflicting torture during interrogation of a suspect, consisting of the victim tied to an inclining board, repeatedly being immersed in water simulating drowning but not allowing to drown, extending the suffering, inciting mortal fear and psychological breakdown. A cruel, unlawful practice against all Red Cross and humane principles and human rights.
Cf. torture, Universal Declaration of Human Rights

Wave Agitation of the surface of the sea caused by local winds. The numerical code representing the state of the sea is the Douglas scale.
Sn: surge
Cf. Douglas scale, tsunami

Wave-generating area Oceanic surface upon which winds blow in constant direction and force.
Cf. force, wind, wind force

Weapons of mass destruction/ WMD Offensive weapons whose destructive capability is derived from nuclear, chemical or biological sources. Sometimes referred to as ABC: atomic, biological, chemical. Their use is prohibited by UN and other international conventions. WMDs are the opposite of conventional arms/weapons.
Cf. biological warfare, chemical warfare, nuclear weapons, conventional arms

Weather forecast Announcement of meteorological conditions anticipated for a specific area and period of time. Weather forecasting is important in disaster prevention and climatological forecast.
Cf. cyclone warning, meteorology, climatological forecast

Weather map Topographic map on which the national meteorological services record data – temperature, humidity, winds, nebulosity, pressure, etc. – every six hours, using symbols, isobars, etc.
Cf. meteorology, topography, climate change

Welfare A general state of a person's or community's satisfaction, health, prosperity, well-being and social support.
Cf. well-being, health, welfare state

Welfare state A nation or state, like the United Kingdom, that provides free health coverage and social services for its entire population – "from cradle to grave" – irrespective of age, wealth or other status.
Cf. welfare, health, national health service, society

Well-being The physical and psychological state that makes an individual feel adjusted to his environment. Also, well being.

Cf. environment, health, needs, World Health Organization

Wheat-soya blend Nutritive food mixture consisting of:
73.1% wheat, precooked
20.0% soya flour
4.0% salad oil, stabilized
2.9% vitamin and mineral premix
Sn: WSB
Cf. food mixtures

Wheat-soya-milk Wheat-soya mixture prepared in milk.
Sn: WSM
Cf. food mixtures

Whirlwind A small scale rotating column of air.
Sn: twister
Cf. tornado

Whistleblower A person in a group, establishment or government who, openly or anonymously, discloses to the public or someone in authority alleged misconduct, fraud, covert or illegal activities in an organization or government. May be damaging or beneficial.
Cf. accountability, transparency, WikiLeaks

WHO Essential Medicines List Cf. Essential medicines

WHO pandemic alert phases/ degrees WHO has a system of six phases for assessing the gravity of an impending major epidemic or pandemic and informing health authorities to take the necessary measures, e.g. in a situation of a new virus A(H1N1) porcine influenza. The decision to pass from one phase to the other and to take the necessary steps is the prerogative of the director general, upon consultation and expert advice.
Phase 1: Small risk of human cases, when there is presence of the virus in animals but not in man.

Phase 2: Slightly elevated risk, with appearance of a few human cases.

Phase 3: The virus starts causing human cases, but not extensively. Early pandemic alert.

Phase 4: Increasing man-to-man transmission. There is risk of a pandemic, but not inevitable.

Phase 5: Heavy man-to-man transmission. High risk of a potential pandemic. The infection has foci in more than two countries of the region. There is little time left to be prepared.

Phase 6: Sustained man-to-man transmission. As of this phase, there is pandemic due to the new dangerous virus. This is officially declared immediately upon noting the presence of the infection in at least two distinct regions in the world – After WHO.

Cf. pandemic, epidemic, A(H1N1) virus

Whooping cough A common, highly infectious communicable disease of childhood characterized by paroxysmal coughing. A significant cause of death in infants in developing countries. Easily preventable and included in the WHO programme of immunization.

Sn: pertussis

Cf. Expanded Programme on Immunization

WHOPAX Report Abridged designation for the Report of the WHO Management Group on the Role of Physicians and Other Health Workers in the Preservation and Promotion of Peace, published under the title "Effects of Nuclear War on Health and Health Services". It concludes that "the only approach to the treatment of health effects…is the prevention of nuclear war".

Cf. World Health Organization, nuclear war, GLAWARS Report

WikiLeaks A not-for-profit, non-governmental organization founded with the purpose of assuring transparency in governmental and international actions by whistle-blowing, retrieving, exposing and publishing diplomatic, secret, private and classified information that concerns society.

Wikipedia A valuable, extensive and varied source of online encyclopaedic information that can be accessed free electronically by anyone. Very useful by its coverage. Can be particularly helpful in the field, remote or disaster site when compiling records or completing reports under conditions where normal sources and reference facilities are not available.

Wildfire Any fire occurring on wildland, of any source, except a fire under prescription – After FAO.

Sn: wildland fire

Willy-willy The Australian term for a tropical cyclone.

Cf. tropical cyclone

Wind Air movement relative to the earth's surface. Unless otherwise specified, only the horizontal component of the movement is considered. The coding of wind velocity is shown by the Beaufort scale.

Cf. Beaufort scale

Wind erosion Erosion of the land due to the action of winds.

Sn: aeolian erosion

Cf. erosion, soil erosion, wind, anthropic erosion

Wind force Force exerted by the wind on a building, plantation, object, etc.

Windhoek Declaration Formal declaration on the freedom of the press, made in 1991, based on the Universal Declaration of Human Rights and endorsed in 1993, calling for free,

independent, pluralistic media worldwide, characterizing free press as a fundamental right.
Cf. freedom of the press

Windscale accident Site of a military nuclear facility in England. On 10 October 1957, the annealing of the graphite moderator at this air-cooled reactor caused the graphite and uranium to catch fire, releasing radioactive material into the atmosphere; important accident rated level 5 on the INES.
Cf. nuclear accident, International Nuclear Event Scale, Sellafield, Mayak, La Hague

Winter blizzard Very cold snowy weather, characterized by strong winds, cold snowy conditions and low visibility. Officially to qualify as w.b., the following are required: (a) temperature at least −12 °C, (b) winds of minimum 40 km/h, (c) visibility less than 1 km and (d) these must last for at least 3 h.
Cf. blizzard, wind

Winter monsoon Continental monsoon which blows in the winter.
Cf. monsoon, summer monsoon

Workshop (educational) An organized series of training sessions that emphasizes free discussion and exchange of ideas, interacting concepts, skills and methods for problem solving and professional development.

World Association for Disaster and Emergency Medicine/WADEM Major worldwide organization of professionals from a wide range of health disciplines engaged in or promoting better knowledge and practice of all aspects of emergency medicine and disaster management. Publisher of "Prehospital and Disaster Medicine".
Cf. disaster medicine, International Association for Humanitarian Medicine

World Bank – IBRD More formally called the International Bank for Reconstruction and Development, a specialized agency of the United Nations set up for economic development, particularly in those two purposes. Also concerned with the interrelationships of health, social development, poverty and globalization.
Cf. sustainable development, health, United Nations, Copenhagen Declaration

World Commission on Environment and Development/Rio The Commission that organized the international "Our Common Future" meeting in Rio in 1987 on policies concerning the environment and development and established the now classic concept of sustainable development.
Cf. sustainable development, development, WCED, MDGs

World Council of Churches/WCC Fellowship of some 300 Christian, mainly non-Catholic churches to promote the unity of the Church and mankind. Active in international affairs with particular attention to conflict situations, human rights, peace, ethics and disaster assistance.
Sn: Oecumenical Council, WCC
Cf. non-governmental organization

World Family Organization Important social NGO in particular upholding women's and family values and health in development. Part of the UN-NGO-IRENE network.

World Federalist Movement/WFM An organization of citizens worldwide that advocates global government, just governance and development of a global community based on practical rule of law, democratically accountable to international institutions. Strives for non-violent improvement of international relations and a more just UN.

World Food Programme/WFP The organization of the United Nations system for food aid, both for development projects and emergency relief in drought or famine, by mobilization of bulk foodstuffs (while FAO mobilizes resources). Has a food-for-work mechanism for refugee and disaster situations.

Sn: WFP

Cf. drought, food aid, Food and Agriculture Organization, United Nations

World Health Organization/WHO The health arm of the United Nations aiming at "the attainment by all peoples of the highest possible level of health" as a human right. Coordinates efforts to raise health levels worldwide and promotes the development of primary health care. Besides multiple public health programmes and actions, it is engaged in disaster preparedness and humanitarian relief both at headquarters and at six Regional Offices and coordinates the health sector of any UN involvement in major emergencies. Has compiled the Emergency Health Kit. Eradicated smallpox.

Sn: WHO

Cf. Emergency Health Kit, primary health care, public health, United Nations, WHOPAX Report, International Association for Humanitarian Medicine Brock Chisholm (Note: Dr. Chisholm was the first director general of WHO.)

World Institute for Development Economics Research/UNU-WIDER World Institute for Development Economics Research, the development study arm of the United Nations University. (Cf.)

World Medical Association/WMA Worldwide federation of the principal medical associations that represent physicians. It works to ensure the independence of the medical profession and is concerned with medical ethics, medical education, socio-medical affairs, rights of the patient and health legislation. With WHO, it formulated the International Code of Medical Ethics.

Cf. bioethics, Nuremberg

World Meteorological Organization/WMO UN specialized agency that promotes the effective use worldwide of meteorological and hydrological information, especially in weather forecasting, water resource prediction and climatology.

A priority function is to oversee the World Weather Watch and World Climate Programme. Important and active in the meteorological aspects of disaster management.

Sn: WMO

Cf. meteorology, World Weather Watch, United Nations

World Open Hospitals/WOH An expanding worldwide voluntary network of hospitals in which the hospital authorities as well as practicing physicians have undertaken to receive and treat without charge, on a purely humanitarian basis, patients from developing countries or disaster areas where the necessary specialized care is lacking or cannot be delivered adequately. Founded by the International Association for Humanitarian Medicine Brock Chisholm.

Sn: WOH

Cf. humanitarian, humanitarian medicine, international assistance, International Association for Humanitarian Medicine

**World Summit for Social Develop-
ment** Cf. Copenhagen Declaration

World Vision International Major
international humanitarian non-
governmental organization widely
present in needy areas for relief and
development. Active in assistance in
disasters and conflicts, promotes
health education in and support for
indigenous populations.
Cf. development, international assistance, indigenous, primary health care

World Weather Watch The global
system of the World Meteorological
Organization for observing, monitoring and exchanging meteorological
information in real time through satellite and other advanced data collecting methods.
Sn: WWW
Cf. satellite, World Meteorological
Organization

X

X-rays Electromagnetic rays, same as
gamma rays, but produced in processes outside the atomic nucleus.
Sn: Roentgen rays

Xenophobia Dread, dislike or hatred of
and opposition to foreigners or ethnic
groups. It is an unacceptable discrimination, against human rights.
Cf. discrimination, human rights

Xenotransplantation Transplanting or
grafting in a person a tissue or organ
that has been derived from a species
different from the recipient.

Xerophthalmia A serious eye disease
due to the total ocular syndrome
associated with vitamin A deficiency,
causing lens opacification, kerato-
malacia and night blindness.
Cf. vitamin A deficiency

Y

Yam Tropical edible plant, the roots of
which are rich in starch and constitute
the staple food in certain regions.
Cf. conventional food, staple food

Yaws A treponemal disease akin to
pinta.
Cf. pinta

**Years Lost due to Disability/
YLDs** Years lost due to disability
are calculated as the number of incident cases × average duration of the
diseases × weight factor to account
for severity – WHO.

Yellow cake Following purification of
uranium 235 by removing the soil
gangue, the resulting concentrate is a
yellow powder, U308, also known as
yellow cake, used for civilian and
military purposes.
Cf. uranium

Yellow fever A highly contagious, acute,
lethal viral disease of Africa and South
America, transmitted by the *Aedes*
mosquito. Death is due to liver and
kidney failure. One of the few remaining quarantinable diseases, successfully preventable by vaccination.
Cf. endemic, epidemic, jaundice,
quarantine

Yoghourt A nutritious, easily digest-
ible, inexpensive dairy product, primarily based on curdled milk, suitable
as nutrition in camps and for the
physically ill.
Also yaourt, yogurt

Yokohama Strategy World Conference
on Natural Disaster Reduction, 1994,
in Yokohama, Japan, promoting the
UN International Decade for Disaster
Reduction 1990–2000 and establishing strategies for a safer world.
Cf. IDNDR, ISDR, OCHA, Hyogo

Z

Zaschita Russian word for protection, the name of the All-Russian Centre for Disaster Medicine (ARCDM). Major governmental facility in Moscow for research, prevention, education and response in disaster medicine.

A WHO Collaborating Centre

Zero option The possibility of agreement between the nuclear powers to reduce the stockpiles of long-range nuclear missiles to nil. Double-zero applies to long-range and medium-range missiles.

Cf. nuclear war, WHOPAX, missiles

Zone Zero/ZZ In a disaster, the immediate area of maximum impact is the epicentre, Ground Zero. A further area of great damage, but less than at the epicentral GZ, surrounds this, with considerable but less destruction and where danger, search-and-rescue, exclusions and restrictions still apply. This secondary area is Zone Zero (ZZ). Example: In the Fukushima disaster, Ground Zero was the area immediately around the damaged reactors, about 5 km. Beyond that, over a perimeter of 20 km, extends Zone Zero – Gunn.

Cf. Fukushima, epicentre, ground zero, Chernobyl

Zonation/Microzoning The division and subdivision of a geographical area – country, region, etc. – and mapping into sectors that are homogeneous with respect to given criteria, microzoning, e.g. according to population density, or a perceived use, resource, hazard, avalanche, seismic fault, flooding or other degrees of risk. It also includes regulations according to each zone or microzone. Also zonation, hazard mapping, resource mapping.

Cf. risk map

Zoonosis Any disease of animals that can be transmitted to man. Examples: rabies, yellow fever, dengue, foot-and-mouth disease, mad cow disease.

Cf. dengue, rabies, yellow fever, bovine spongiform encephalopathy, BSE, Creutzfeldt-Jakob disease, epizootic

Part II
Acronyms and Abbreviations

An asterisk (*) refers to this term in Part I, the Dictionary

A

AAA *Accra Agenda for Action

AAH Action Against Hunger

AAM Air-to-air *missile

AB *Atom bomb, *atomic bomb

ABC Airway, breathing, circulation (emergency medicine)
Atomic, biological, chemical (weapons)

ABM *Antiballistic missile

ABU Asia-Pacific Broadcasting Union

AC Arctic Council

ACC Administrative Committee on Coordination (United Nations)

ACF Action Contre la Faim (Action Against Hunger: AAH)

ACGHST African Centre for Global Health and Social Transformation

ACHPR African Charter on Human and Peoples' Rights

ACLS *Advanced cardiac life support

ACORD Agency for Cooperation and Research in Development

ACS *American College of Surgeons

ACSM Advocacy, communication and social mobilization

ACT Action by Churches Together

ACTED Artemisinin-based combination therapy (against malaria)
Agency for Technical Cooperation and Development

ACUNS *Academic Council on the United Nations System

ADB African Development Bank

AsDB Asian Development Bank

ADI Acceptable daily intake (of toxic substance)

ADP Asian Disaster Preparedness Center (AIT)

ADRA Adventist Development and Relief Agency

AERE Atomic Energy Research Establishment (UK – Harwell)

AEROSAT International Aeronautic Satellite Programme

AFB Acid-fast bacilli

AFP Agence France Presse

AFRO Regional Office for Africa (WHO)

AFY Advocates for Youth

AGBU Armenian General Benevolent Union

AGFUND Arab Gulf Fund for United Nations Development

AGM Air-to-ground *missile

A(H1N1) Porcine influenza virus strain
*Swine influenza virus pandemic 2009

AHCO AIDS Healthcare Organization

AHH Arbeitsstab Humanitäre Hilfe (Germany)

AHPSR Alliance for Health Policy and Systems Research (WHO)

S.W.A. Gunn, *Dictionary of Disaster Medicine and Humanitarian Relief*,
DOI 10.1007/978-1-4614-4445-9_2, © Springer Science+Business Media New York 2013

AI *Amnesty International

AID United States Agency for International Development (also USAID)

AIDES Italian association for health development

*__AIDS/Aids__ *Acquired immunodeficiency syndrome (also HIV/AIDS)

AIFOMD Association Internationale de Formateurs en Objectifs du Millénaire pour le Développement / IAMDGT

AIS Abbreviated injury scale

AIT Asian Institute of Technology

AIUTA Association Internationale des Universités du Troisième Age

AKF *Aga Khan Foundation

*__ALARA__ *As low as reasonably achievable (radiation dose)

ALDHU Latin American Human Rights Association

ALITE Augmented Logistics Intervention Team (WFP)

*__ALS__ *Advanced life support (anaesthesia, emergency)

AM Transmission through amplitude modulation

AMA American Medical Association

AMAP Arctic Monitoring Assessment Programme

AMDF AIDS-adjusted PMDF

AMELISAP Association des Médecins Libéraux Sapeurs Pompiers

AMI Acute myocardial infarction

AMP Agence de Médecine Préventive

AMPATH Academic Model for Prevention and Treatment of HIV/AIDS

AmRC/ARC American Red Cross

*__AMRO__ Regional Office for the Americas (WHO)

AMSAT Amateur satellite

AMVER Automated Mutual Assistance Vessel Rescue

ANC Antenatal care
African National Congress (South Africa)

AP Associated Press

*__APACHE__ *Acute physiology and chronic health evaluation

APCDM *Asia-Pacific Conference on Disaster Medicine

API Active pharmaceutical ingredient

APM Asociaciòn Abuelas de Plaza de Mayo (Association of Grandmothers of Plaza de Mayo – Argentina)

APOC African Programme for Onchocerciasis Control (WHO)

APPS African Partnership for Public Health Safety

APT *Association for the Prevention of Torture

APU *Auxiliary power unit

ARABSAT Arab Satellite Communications Organization

ARC American Refugee Committee

ARCDM All-Russian Centre for Disaster Medicine *Zaschita

ARD *Acute respiratory disease (or distress)

ARI Annual risk of infection

ARPCT Alliance for Restoration of Peace and Counter-Terrorism

ARSI *Association of Rural Surgeons of India

ART Antiretroviral therapy

ARV Antiretrovirus

ASAFED African Association of Education for Development

ASAP As soon as possible

ASEAN Association of Southeast Asian Nations

ASH Action on Smoking and Health

ASI Anti-Slavery International

ATA Actual time of arrival

ATD Actual time of departure

ATLS *Advanced trauma life support

ATOP *Association for Trauma Outreach and Prevention

ATTAC *Attac. (French): Association pour une Taxation des Transactions financières pour l'Aide aux Citoyens

ATWC Alaska *Tsunami Warning Center

AU African Union (previously OAU: Organization of African Unity)

AVPU *Awake, verbal response, pain response, unresponsive

AVSI Association of Volunteers in International Service

AWACS Airborne Warning and Control System

AWRE Atomic Weapons Research Establishment

B

BAL British anti-lewisite

BBC British Broadcasting Corporation

*BCG *Bacille Calmette-Guérin (anti-TB vaccine)

BCT (WHO Department of) Blood Safety and Clinical Technology

BDP Bureau for Development Policy (UNDP)

BDS *Bradford Disaster Scale

BENELUX Belgium, the Netherlands, Luxembourg

BHR Bureau for Humanitarian Response (US-OFDA)

*BLEVE *Boiling liquid expanded vapour explosion

BLS *Basic life support

BMA British Medical Association

BMI Body mass index

BMR *Basal metabolic rate

BMS Breast milk substitute

BOD *Burden of disease

BP Medicine: Blood pressure
Industry: British Petroleum

*Bq *Becquerel (unit of nuclear activity that has replaced the curie)

BRICS Brazil, Russia, India, China, South Africa (major emerging countries)

*BSA *Body surface area (of burn injury)

BSE *Bovine spongiform encephalopathy (mad cow disease)

BTS *Blood transfusion service

BW *Biological warfare/biological weapon(s)

BWC *Biological Weapons Convention

C

°C Celsius (degree of heat; has replaced the centigrade)

C³ Command, control and communications

CAD Coronary artery disease

CAF Cost and freight

CAFOD Catholic Fund for Overseas Development

cal Calorie (unit of heat)

CALD Culturally and linguistically diverse

CARE Cooperative for Assistance and Relief Everywhere

CARICOM Caribbean Community and Common Market

*CARITAS *International Confederation of Catholic Organizations for Charitable and Social Action

CARTA Consortium for Advanced Research Training in Africa

CAS Collision avoidance system

CASs Country assistance strategies

CASA Coordinating Action on Small Arms

CAT *Convention Against Torture and Other Cruel, Inhuman or Degrading Treatment or Punishment

CATW Coalition Against Trafficking in Women

CBC Community-based care

CBD Canadian Broadcasting Corporation

CBJO Coordinating Board of Jewish Organizations

CBO Community-based organization

CBRN Chemical, biological, radiological, nuclear, (non-conventional weapons)

cc Cubic centimetre

CC Corps Consulaire/Consular Corps

CCCF Canadian Child Care Federation (FCSGE)

CCD Convention to Combat Desertification (UN)

CCF Christian Children's Fund

CCIA Commission of the Churches on International Affairs

CCS *Casualty Clearing Station Country Cooperation Strategy (WHO)

CCW Convention on Prohibitions or Restrictions on the Use of Certain Conventional Weapons which may be Deemed to be Excessively Injurious or to have Indiscriminate Effects

CD Conference on Disarmament Corps Diplomatique/Diplomatic Corps

CDC Centers for Disease Control and Prevention (USA)

CDCIR Community Documentation Centre on Industrial Risk

CDE Centre International de l'Enfance (ICC, Paris)

CE Council of Europe/Conseil de l'Europe

CECP Committee Encouraging Corporate Philanthropy

CEDAW Convention on the Elimination of All Forms of Discrimination Against Women

CEF Central Emergency Response Fund

CEMD Confidential enquiry into maternal deaths

CEMEC *European Centre for Disaster Medicine/Centro Europeo per la Medicina delle Catastrofi

CEPREDENAC Centro de Prevenciòn para Desastres Naturales en America Central

CERD Committee on the Elimination of Racial Discrimination (UN)

CERF Central Emergency Response Fund

CERN Centre Européen pour la Recherche Nucléaire–European Centre for Nuclear Research

CESCR Committee on Economic, Social and Cultural Rights (UN)

CETIM *Centre Europe – Tiers Monde

CFC *Chemistry: chlorofluorocarbons UN: Common Fund for Commodities

CFR Case fatality rate

CFS Committee on World Food Security

CFSAM Crop and Food Supply Assessment Mission (WFP-FAO)

CGF Calouste *Gulbenkian Foundation

CHAP Common Humanitarian Action Plan Consolidated Humanitarian Assistance Programme

CHD Child Health and Development (Division of WHO)

CHF Canadian Hunger Foundation

CHH Child-headed household

CHOICE-WHO CHOosing Interventions that are Cost Effective-WHO

CHP Centre for Humanitarian Psychology

CHW *Community health worker

CI *Caritas Internationalis (CARITAS) Conservation International

CIA Central Intelligence Agency (USA)

CICARWS Commission on Inter-Church Aid, Refugee and World Service

CICP Centre for International Crime Prevention

CICR/ICRC *Comité International de la Croix-Rouge – International Committee of the Red Cross

CICRED Committee for International Cooperation in National Research in Demography

CIDA *Canadian International Development Agency

CIHC Center for International Health and Cooperation

CIHR Canadian Institutes of Health Research

CIGLOB International Center for Globalization and Development

CIF Cost, insurance and freight

CILSS Permanent Interstate Committee for Drought Control in the *Sahel

CIM Committee for International *Migration

CIMIC Civilian-military cooperation

CINDI Children in Distress International

CIOMS Council for International Organizations of Medical Sciences

CIPIH Commission on Intellectual Property Rights, Innovation and Public Health (WHO)

CISFAM Consolidated Information System for *Famine Management in Africa

CISP Comitato Internazionale per lo Sviluppo dei Popoli

CISR Center for International Stabilization and Recovery (of *landmines)

CITES Convention on International Trade in Endangered Species of Wild Fauna and Flora

CIVICUS World Alliance for Citizen Participation

CLAS Culturally and linguistically appropriate health services

cm Centimetre

CMA *Cranfield Mine Action Canadian Medical Association

CMH Commission on Macroeconomics and Health (WHO)

CMI Crop moisture index

CMR Crude mortality rate

CND Campaign for Nuclear Disarmament

CNN Cable News Network

CNS Central nervous system

CO₂ *Carbon dioxide

COC Combined oral contraceptive

COD Cash on delivery

COHRED *Council on Health Research for Development

COMPAS Commodity Movement Processing and Analysis System (WFP)

COMSAT Communications Satellite Corporation

CONGO Conference of Non-Governmental Organizations in Consultative Status with the United Nations Economic and Social Council

COPD Chronic obstructive pulmonary disease

COR UNUM Coordination of Roman Catholic Relief Agencies

COSECSA College of Surgeons of East, Central and Southern Africa

COSME Operational Coordination of Medical Emergencies Surveillance (Italy)

COVAW Coalition on *Violence Against Women

CPI/TI *Corruption Perceptions Index of Transparency International

CpiE Child Protection in Emergencies

CPR *Cardiopulmonary resuscitation

CR (E) Casualty rate (estimation)

CRC Committee on the Rights of the Child

***CRED** *Centre for Research on the Epidemiology of Disasters (Belgium)

CRS Catholic Relief Services

CSB *Corn-soya blend

CSD Commission on *Sustainable Development

CSIRO Commonwealth Scientific and Industrial Research Organization (Australia)

CSM *Corn-soya milk

CSO Civil Service Organization

CSOPP Civil Society Organizations and Participation Programme (UNDP)

CSOU *Civil Society and Outreach Unit (UN-DSPD)

CSR Corporate social responsibility

CSW Commercial sex worker

CTBT Comprehensive Nuclear-Test-Ban Treaty

CTBTO Comprehensive Nuclear-Test-Ban-Treaty Organization

CTS Communications Technology Satellite

CTV Centre for Torture Victims (Bosnia-Herzegovina)

CUI *Chernobyl Union International

CUSO Canadian University Services Overseas

CVA *Cerebrovascular accident

CVD Cardiovascular disease

CVM Complex of vitamins and minerals

CW *Chemical warfare/chemical weapon

CWC *Chemical Weapons Convention

CWGL Center for Women's Global Leadership

CWS Church World Service

D

DAC Development Assistance Committee (OECD)

DALE *Disability-adjusted life expectancy

DALY(s) *Disability-adjusted life year(s)

DANIDA Danish International Development Agency

DARA *Development Assistance Research Associates

DART Disaster Assistance Response Team (US/AID and Canada)

DAW Division for the Advancement of Women (UN)

DBS Direct broadcast satellite

DCCP Disaster critical control point

DCI Defence of Children International/ DEI: Défense des Enfants International

DCF Development Cooperation Forum

DDA Department of Disarmament Affairs (UN)

DDD Direct distance dialling

DDR Disarmament, demobilization and reintegration

DDT Dichlorodiphenyltrichloroethane (insecticide)

DDW Das Diakonische Werk – German church service

DECAF *Democratic Control of Armed Forces/Geneva

DECIPHer Centre for the Development and Evaluation of Complex Interventions for Public Health Improvement

DELNET Development local network (*ILO)

DESA Department of Economic and Social Affairs (UN)

DEW Distant Early Warning (military radar network)

DFCM *Dried full-cream milk

DFID Department for Foreign International Development (UK)

DHA *UN Department of Humanitarian Affairs (see OCHA)

DHD *Disaster health diplomacy

DHS Demographic and health surveys

DIANE Direct Information Access Network for Europe

*DNA *Deoxyribonucleic acid

DNDi *Drugs for Neglected Diseases initiative

DNR Do not resuscitate

DOA/d.o.a. Dead on arrival

DoC Declaration of commitment

DOC Direct operating costs

DoCip Documentation Centre for Indigenous Peoples' Research and Information

DOTS Directly observed treatment short course (for TB, WHO)

DP Displaced person(s)

DPA Department of Political Affairs (UN)

DPI Department of Public Information/ UN

Disabled Peoples' International

DPKO *UN Department of Peace-keeping Operations

DPLU Disaster Prevention and Limitation Unit (*Bradford University, UK)

DPT *Diphtheria-pertussis-tetanus (vaccine)

DRC Danish Refugee Council

DRK Deutsches Rotes Kreuz (German Red Cross)

DRS Drug resistance surveillance (or survey)

DRSE Drug-related side effects

DSA Daily subsistence allowance

DSM *Dried skim milk

DSPD Division of Social Policy and Development (UN-DESA)

DWH Deutsche Welthungerhilfe (German hunger aid)

DWM *Dried whole milk

E

EAC East African Community

EAFORD International Organization for the Elimination of All Forms of Racial Discrimination

EBM Evidence-based medicine

EBU/UER European Broadcasting Union/Union Européenne de Radiodiffusion

EDM (WHO Department of) Essential Drugs and Medicines Policy

EC European Commission

ECA Economic Commission for Africa

ECB European Central Bank

ECDC European Centre for Disease Prevention and Control

ECE Economic Commission for Europe

ECFMG Educational Council for Foreign Medical Graduates (USA)

ECHO*European Community Humanitarian Office (EU)

ECHUI Ending Child Hunger and Undernutrition Initiative

ECLAC Economic Commission for Latin America and the Caribbean (UN)

ECLS Extracorporeal life support

ECOSOC Economic and Social Council of the United Nations

ECOWAS Economic Community of West African States

ECP Essential clinical package

ECPAT End Child Prostitution in Asian Tourism International

ECWA Economic Commission for Western Asia

ED/EM Essential drugs/essential medicines

EFA Education for All

EFNA Emergency Food Needs assessment

EHA Emergency and Humanitarian Action (WHO)

*eHealth Electronic health

EHESS L'Ecôle de Hautes Etudes en Sciences Sociales

EHRP Emergency Humanitarian Response Plan

EIA Environmental impact assessment

EMERCOM Emergency Committee (Russia)

EMMIR Emergency military medical assistance (France)

EMOP Emergency operation

EMP *Electromagnetic pulse

EMRIP UN Expert Mechanism on the Rights of Indigenous Peoples

EMRO Regional Office for the Eastern Mediterranean (WHO)

EMS *Emergency medical services

ENEA (Italian Committee for) Nuclear Energy and Alternative Energies

ENSO *El Ninô – Southern Oscillation (meteorology)

EOC Emergency operations centre

EOE Equal opportunity employer

EPA Environmental Protection Agency (USA)

EPGH European Partnership in Global Health

EPHI Essential Public Health Interventions

EPI *Expanded Programme on Immunization (WHO-UNICEF)

EPRP Emergency Preparedness and Response Plan

EPSCO Employment, Social Policy, and Health and Consumer Affairs Council

EQA External quality assessment

ERC Emergency Relief Coordinator – UN New York

ER&FS Early Recovery and Food Security work plan

ERM *Emergency Risk Management and Humanitarian Response (WHO) (previously HAC and ERO)

ERNA Early Recovery Needs Assessment

ERTS Earth Resources Technology Satellite

ESA European Space Agency

ESCAP Economic and Social Commission for Asia and the Pacific (UN)

ESPRIT European Strategic Programme for Research and Development in Information Technology

ETA Expected time of arrival

ETD Expected time of departure

ETR Expected time of return

EU European Union

EURO/Euro Regional Office for Europe (WHO)

The European currency unit

Expat Expatriate person

F

°F Degree Fahrenheit

FAAD Food Aid and Development (WFP policies)

F&D/f&d Commerce: Freight and demurrage

FAO *Food and Agriculture Organization / UN

f.a.q. Commerce/shipping: Free alongside quay

FAR *Fund for Armenian Relief

FAS Commerce/shipping: Free alongside ship

FAWE Forum for African Women Educationalists

FBF *Fortified blended food

FBI Federal Bureau of Investigation (USA)

Focal brain ischaemia

FBO Faith-based organization

FCM *Full cream milk powder

FDA Food and Drug Administration (USA)

FDC Fixed-dose combination

FDI Foreign direct investment

*Fédération Dentaire Internationale/ WDF

FERI Franklin and Eleanor Roosevelt Institute

FFH/CAFD Freedom From Hunger – Campaign Action For Development

FFR Food for recovery

FFW Food for work

FGM *Female genital mutilation

FHI Food for the Hungry International

FHR Medicine: foetal heart rate

FICSA Former International Civil Servants' Association (UN)

FIDH International Federation for Human Rights

FIGO Fédération Internationale de Gynécologie et Obstétrique

FIND *Foundation for Innovative New Diagnostics

FMEA Failure mode and effects analysis (also HC-FMEA)

FOB Commerce: free on board

f.o.s. Commerce: free on ship

f.o.t. Commerce: free of tax

FPC Fish protein concentrate

FPIC Free, prior and informed consent

ft Foot or feet (measure)

FXBI *Association François-Xavier Bagnoud/FXB International

FYI/f.y.i. For your information

G

g Gram or gramme

G8 Group of eight leading rich industrial countries

G20 *Group of 20 leading rich industrial countries

G77 Group of 77 developing, non-aligned countries

GAA German Agro Action

GACD Global Alliance for Chronic Diseases

GAIN *Global Alliance for Improved Nutrition

GAINS Gender Awareness Information and Networking System

gal Gallon

GARP Global Atmosphere Research Programme

GAVI *Global Alliance for Vaccines and Immunization

GBD Global burden of disease

GBV Gender-based violence

GCCA Global Climate Change Alliance

GCI *Green Cross International

GCIM Global Commission on International Migration

GCS *Glasgow Coma Scale

GCSF Global *Civil Society Forum

GDA Global Development Alliance (USAID)

GDF Global Drug Facility (e.g. against tuberculosis)

GDP/gdp Gross domestic product

GenCap Gender Standby Capacity Project

*GEO Group on Earth Observations

GFAT *Global Fund to Fight AIDS, Tuberculosis and Malaria (also GF)

GFHR *Global Forum for Health Research

GFMER Geneva Foundation for Medical Education and Research

GFR General fertility rate

GH *Global health

GHC/WHO *Global Health Cluster/WHO

GHD *Global health diplomacy *Good Humanitarian Donorship

GHF Geneva Health Forum

GHG (Global) *greenhouse gas

GHP Global Health Partnership (WHO)

GHWA Global Health Workforce Alliance

GIAN Geneva International Academic Network

GIEESC *Global Initiative for Emergency and Essential Surgical Care (WHO)

GIIDS *Graduate Institute of International and Development Studies (Graduate Institute, Geneva)

GINA Geneva International Network on Ageing

GIPRI Geneva International Peace Research Institute

GIS Geographic information systems

GISAH Global Information System on Alcohol and Health

GIVS Global Immunization Vision and Strategy

GLI Global Laboratory Initiative

Global Fund *Global Fund to Fight Aids, Tuberculosis and Malaria

GLOBE Global Legislators Organization for a Balanced Environment

GMAD Global Mine Action Directory

GMDS Global Maritime Distress and Safety System

GMEF Global Ministerial Environment Forum

GMF Genetically modified food

GMO Genetically modified organism

GMP/WHO *Good manufacturing practices (WHO model)

GMT Greenwich Mean Time

GNI Gross national income

GNP *Gross national product

GO Governmental organization

GOARN Global Outbreak Alert and Response Network

***GOES** Geostationary Operational Environmental Satellite / *Global-Observing Environmental Satellite

GOS Global Observing System

GPEI Global Polio Eradication Initiative

GPS Global Positioning System

GPSC Global Patient Safety Challenge (WHO)

GRID Global Resource Information Database

GRIPP Global Review and Inventory of Population Policies

GRT Gross register tonnage

GSO Geostationary satellite orbit

Gy *Gray (Unit of radioactive absorbed dose)

H

H1N1 Swine influenza virus strain (*pandemic)

H5N1 *Avian influenza virus strain (*epidemic)

H₂O *Water

HAV *Hepatitis A virus

HABITAT United Nations Centre for Human Settlements (UNCHS)

HAC Health Action in Crises (WHO) (changed to *ERM)

HACCP Hazard Analysis and Critical Control Point system

HALE Health-adjusted life expectancy (see *QALY)

HBC(s) High-burden countries

HBV *Hepatitis B virus

HC-FMEA Health care – failure modes and effects analysis

HCHR *High Commissioner for Human Rights (also OHCHR, UNHCHR)

HCR *High Commissioner for Refugees (also UNHCR)

HDI Human development index

HDR Humanitarian daily *ration

HDS Department of Health Policy, Development and Services (WHO)

HDTC Humanitarian Demining Training Center

HE High energy (food)

HELP Health Emergencies in Large Populations

HEM High-energy milk (feeding mixture)

HFA Hyogo Framework for Action

HHS Health and Human Services Department (USA)

HIC *High-income country

HIID Harvard Institute for International Development

HILAC Heavy-ion linear accelerator

HIPC Heavily indebted poor countries

HiT Health care systems in transition

HIV *Human immunodeficiency virus

HIV/AIDS *Human immunodeficiency disease (also AIDS)

HLF High-Level Forum (on health MDGs)

HPC Hiroshima* Peacebuilders Center (Japan)

HRC Human Rights Council

HRI *Humanitarian Response Index

HRIC UN Office of Human Resources for International Cooperation (DESA)

HRP UNDP/UNFPA/WHO/WB Special Programme of Research, Development and Research Training in Human Reproduction

HRT Hormone replacement therapy

HRW Human Rights Watch

HSP Health sector profile

HSR Health sector reform

HTA Health technology assessment

HUGO Human Genome Organization

HuMA *Humanitarian Medical Assistance (Japan)

HUMV/Humvee Human military light vehicle

HW Hazardous *waste

I

IAEA *International Atomic Energy Agency (UN)

IAESCSI International Association of Economic and Social Councils and Similar Institutions (AICESIS)

IAF International Abolitionist Federation

IAGS International Association of *Genocide Scholars

IAHM *International Association for Humanitarian Medicine Brock Chisholm

IALANA International Association of Lawyers Against Nuclear Arms

IAMANEH *International Association for Maternal and Neonatal Health

IAMDGT/AIFOMD International Association of MDG Trainers/ Association Internationale de Forma- teurs pour les Objectifs du Millénaire du Développement – AIFOMD

IANSA International Action Network on Small Arms

IAPSO International Association for the Physical Sciences of the Oceans

IAR International Association for Religious Freedom

IARF Inter-Agency Procurement Services Office (UNDP)

IAS International Amateur Radio Union International AIDS Society

IASC Inter-Agency Standing Commit- tee for Humanitarian Action

IATA International Air Transport Association

IAVCEI International Association of Volcanology and Chemistry of the Earth's Interior

IAW International Alliance of Women

IBE International Bureau of Education

IBHR *International Bill of Human Rights

IBRD *International Bank for Reconstruction and Development (also *World Bank)

ICAA International Council on Alcohol and Addictions

ICAN International Campaign to Abolish *Nuclear Weapons

ICAO International Civil Aviation Organization (UN)

ICARRD International Conference on Agrarian Reform and Rural Develop- ment

ICBL International Campaign to Ban *Landmines

ICBM Intercontinental ballistic *missile

ICC *International Criminal Court (for war crimes – The Hague)

ICCPR International Covenant on Civil and Political Rights

ICD-10 International Classification of Diseases and Related Health Problems, 10th Revision (WHO) International Statistical Classification of Diseases (WHO)

ICDO *International Civil Defence Organisation

ICECI International Classification of External Causes of Injury (WHO)

ICESCR International Covenant on Economic, Social and Cultural Rights

ICHRN International Centre for Human Resources in Nursing

ICIDH International Classification of Impairments, Disabilities, and Handicaps (WHO)

ICJ *International Court of Justice International Commission of Jurists

ICM Intergovernmental Committee for *Migration

ICMH *International Centre for Migration and Health

ICMC International Catholic Migration Commission

ICN International Council of Nurses

ICPD International Conference on Population and Development

ICPO "Interpol" – International Criminal Police Organization

ICR International Centre of Radio-pathology

ICRC *International Committee of the Red Cross

ICR-DC International Cooperation Research for Developing Countries

ICRP International Commission on Radiological Protection / *IAEA

ICRU International Commission on Radiation Units and Measurements

ICS *Incident Command System

ICSLS International Convention for Safety of Life at Sea

ICSM *Instant corn-soya milk

ICSR International Centre for the Study of Radicalisation and Political Violence

ICSU International Council of Scientific Unions

ICT Information and communications technology

ICTAC International Institute for Counter-Terrorism International Counter-Terrorism Academic Community

ICTR *International Criminal Tribunal for Rwanda

ICTY International Criminal Tribunal for the Former Yugoslavia

ICU *Intensive care unit

ICVA International Council of Voluntary Agencies

ID Identity document International dollar (also I$)

IDA *International Development Association (World Bank Group) Islamic Democratic Association

IDB Inter-American Development Bank

IDDM Insulin-dependent diabetes mellitus

IDP *Internally displaced person

IDRC International Development Research Centre (Canada)

IDRM International Institute for Disaster Risk Management

IDRO International Disaster Relief Operation

IDTR&M Identification, documentation, tracing, reunification and mediation

IDWIP International Decade of the World's Indigenous Peoples

IEA International Energy Agency

IEC International Electrotechnical Commission

IEDD Improvised explosive device disposal

IFAD International Fund for Agricultural Development (UN)

IFCT International Forum for Counter-Terrorism

IFF Identification – friend or foe (radar identity system)

IFFIm International Finance Facility for Immunisation

IFHHRO International Federation of Health and Human Rights Organisations

IFMSA *International Federation of Medical Students' Associations

IFPMA International Federation of Pharmaceutical Manufacturers and Associations

IFRC *International Federation of Red Cross and Red Crescent Societies

IFSC *International Federation of Surgical Colleges

IFUW International Federation of University Women

IGCC Intergovernmental Group on *Climate Change

IGO Intergovernmental organization

IHEID Institut de Hautes Etudes Internationales et du Développement / The *Graduate Institute, Geneva

IHEU International Humanist and Ethical Union

IHF International Hospital Federation

IHL *International humanitarian law

IHR *International Health Regulations (2005)

IIHL International Institute of Humanitarian Law

IISEE International Institute of Seismology and Earthquake Engineering

IIWF International Independent Women's Forum

ILA International Law Association

ILC International Law Commission

ILO *International Labour Organization (UN)

ILOS In-patient length of stay (in hospital)

IMARSAT International Maritime Satellite Organization (also INMARSAT)

IMC International Medical Corps

IMCO International Maritime Consultative Organization (UN)

IMF *International Monetary Fund

IMO International Maritime Organization

IMPACT *International Medical Products Anti-Counterfeiting Taskforce

IMPATT Impact avalanche transit time

IMRA Independent Media Review and Analysis

IMSAR International Maritime Search and Rescue Plan

in Inch

INADES Institut Africain pour le Développement Economique et Social

INCB International Narcotics Control Board

INES *International Nuclear Event Scale

INF Intermediate-Range Nuclear Forces

INFDC International Nutrition Foundation for Developing Countries

INFOTERRA Sources of technical, scientific and decision-oriented information

INMARSAT International Maritime Satellite Organization (also IMARSAT)

INPEA International Network for Prevention of Elder Abuse

INRUD International Network for the Rational Use of Drugs

INSARAG International Search and Rescue Advisory Group

INSTRAW International Research and Training Institute for the Advancement of Women (UN)

INTELSAT International Telecommunications Satellite Consortium

Interpol International Criminal Police Organization (ICPO)

INTERSPUTNIK International Organization of Space Communications

IOM *International Organization for Migration

IPA International Paediatric Association

IPB International Peace Bureau (Geneva)

IPC International Polar Commission

IPCC Intergovernmental Panel on *Climate Change

IPCS *International Programme on Chemical Safety (WHO-UNEP)

IPEC International Programme on the Elimination of Child Labour

IPI International Press Institute

IPO Indigenous peoples' organization

IPPF International Planned Parenthood Federation

IPPNW *International Physicians for the Prevention of Nuclear War

IPRAS International Confederation for Plastic, Reconstructive, and Aesthetic Surgery

IPT Isoniazid preventive therapy
IPU Inter-Parliamentary Union
IPV Inactivated polio vaccine
IRC International Rescue Committee
IRENE Informal Regional Network of NGOs
IRP *International Recovery Platform
IRPTC International Register of Potentially Toxic Chemicals
IRR Incidence rate ratio
IRS Indoor residual spraying
ISBI International Society for Burn Injuries
ISDR *International Strategy for Disaster Reduction (UN)
ISIS International Satellite for Ionospheric Studies
ISO International Organization for Standardization
ISS International Social Service / SSI
ISTC International Standards for Tuberculosis Care
ITACCS International Trauma Anaesthesia Critical Care Society
ITIC International Tsunami Information Center (Honolulu)
ITN Insecticide-treated mosquito net
ITU *International Telecommunication Union (UN)
   Intensive therapy unit (also ICU)
IUD Intra-uterine device (for contraception)
IV (i.v.) Medicine: Intravenous
IWGIA International Working Group for Indigenous Affairs
IWTC International Women's Tribune Centre

J

J joule
JCWI Joint Council for the Welfare of Immigrants

JDR Japan Disaster Relief
JFAM Joint Food Needs Assessment Mission (WFP/UNHCR)
JICA *Japan International Cooperation Agency
JMTDR *Japan Medical Team for Disaster Relief

K

kcal *Kilocalorie (energy unit)
KCSJ Knight Commander of the Order of St. John of Jerusalem (also KSJ, Knights Hospitaller)
***Kerma** Kinetic energy released in matter
KFOR Multinational Kosovo Force
Kg Kilogram (or kilogramme)
KKK Ku Klux Klan (US)
Km *Kilometre or kilometer (also km)
Kt *Kiloton
kw *Kilowatt

L

LA Lead Agency
LANDSAT Earth Resources Technology Satellite
***Laser** Light amplification by stimulated emission of radiation
LAV Light armoured vehicle
lb *Pound
LCT Landing craft tank
LDC *Least-developed countries
LD-50 Median lethal dose
LDF Local development fund
LHRD Lawyers for Human Rights and Development
LIFDC Low-income, food-deficit country
LLITN Long-lasting insecticide-treated net (against malaria). Also LLIN
LMIC Low- and middle-income countries

LPG Liquified petroleum gas

LSHTM London School of Hygiene and Tropical Medicine

LTSH Land-side transport, storage and handling

LWR Lutheran World Relief

LWS Lutheran World Service

M

m *Metre or meter

MAD Military: Mutual   assured destruction

M&E Monitoring and evaluation

MAIC Mine Action Information Center (see ICBL)

MAROTS Maritime orbital test satellite

MARS Major accident reporting system

MASCAL *Mass casualty

MASH Mobile army surgical hospital

MBC *Mediterranean   Council   for Burns and Fire Disasters / *Euro-Mediterranean Council for Burns and Fire Disasters

MCDA Military and civil defence assets

MCH Mother and child health

MCI *Mass casualty incident

MCO Managed care organization

MDG(s) UN Millennium Development Goal(s) *Millennium Development Goal(s)

MDM Médecins du Monde / Doctors of the World

MDTF Multi-donor trust fund

MDR Multidrug resistant disease (see also XDR) Multidrug resistant

MDR-TB Multidrug resistant tuberculosis (with isoniazid and rifampicin resistance)

MDS Maritime Distress and Safety System

MEDICS Medical Information and Coordination System

MEDINT Medical intelligence

MEDLARS Medical   Literature Analysis and Retrieval System

MEDLINE Medical Literature Online (NLM)

MERLIN Medical Emergency Relief International

METEOSAT Meteorological Satellite, Europe

METTAG Medical emergency triage tag Medical Emergency *Triage Tag

MFI *Microfinance institution

*Mg Milligramme or milligram (also mg)

MHI *Major hazard installation

MI5 British counter-intelligence agency

MI6 British intelligence and espionage agency

MIC Methyl   isocyanate   (*Bhopal disaster of 1984)

MIDAS Missile Defense Alarm System

MIM Multilateral Initiative on Malaria (in Africa)

MINURCAT UN Mission in the Central African Republic and Chad

MINUSTAH UN Stabilization Mission in Haiti

MIRV Multiple independently targetable re-entry vehicle

MISP Minimum initial service package

MMEIG Maternal Mortality Estimation Inter-agency Group

MMR Measles-mumps-rubella (vaccine) Maternal mortality rate/ratio

MMI *Medicus Mundi International

MMV Medicines for Malaria Venture

MNT Maternal and neonatal tetanus

MONUC Mission in the Democratic Republic of the Congo (UN)

MOF *Multiple organ failure

MOH Ministry of Health

MOTAPM Explosive remnants of war and mines other than anti-personnel landmines

MoU Memorandum of understanding

MRI Magnetic resonance imaging (body scan)

MRSA Methicillin-resistant *Staphylococcus aureus*

MSAC *Most seriously affected countries

MSF *Médecins sans Frontières / Doctors Without Borders

MSH Management sciences for health

MSW Medical social worker

Mt *Megaton

MT Metric tonne

MTA *Medicines Transparency Alliance

MTE Mass toxicological event

MTF Medical treatment facility

MUAC Medicine: Mid-upper-arm circumference

MW Megawatt

N

NAICC National   Aborigine   and Islander Child Care (Australia)

*Napalm Aluminium naphthenate – aluminium palmitite (weapon)

NASA National Aeronautics and Space Administration (USA)

NATO *North   Atlantic   Treaty Organization

Nazi (German): Nazional-sozialisten

NC Nuremberg Charter

NCBW Nuclear, chemical and biological warfare (or weapon)

NCD Noncommunicable disease

NCHS National   Centre   for   Health Statistics

NDP National drug policy

NFI Non-food item

NFZ Nuclear-free zone

NGLS *United   Nations   Non-Governmental Liaison Service

NGO *Non-governmental organization

NGS Nuclear generating station

NHDP National Health Development Plan

NHS National Health Service

NIH Nationl Institutes of Health

NIS Newly Independent State(s)

NNHT Nuffield Nursing Homes Trust (UK)

NNT Nuclear Non-prolferation Treaty (also NPT)

NOAA National   Oceanic   and Atmospheric Administration

NORAD Norwegian   Agency   for Development Cooperation

North   American   Air   Defense Command

NPA Norwegian Peoples' Aid

NPC National Programme Coordinator (WHO)

*NPT Treaty on the Non-Proliferation of Nuclear Weapons

NRC Nuclear Regulatory Commission (US)

NRDS Neonatal   respiratory   distress syndrome

NRO National Reconnaissance Office (USA)

*NRT Net registered tonnage

NTD *Neglected tropical disease(s)

NTP National tuberculosis control programme (or equivalent)

NWC National   WHO   Programme Coordinator

NWFZ Nuclear-weapons-free zone

NYD Medicine: Not yet diagnosed

O

OAS Organization of American States

OAU Organization of African Unity. (Changed to AU: African Union)

OCHA *Office for the Coordination of Humanitarian Affairs (UN)

ODA Official development assistance Overseas Development Agency

ODCCP Office for Drug Control and Crime Prevention / UN

ODI Overseas Development Institute (UK)

OECD Organization for Economic Cooperation and Development

OFDA *Office of Foreign Disaster Assistance (USA)

OHA Office for Humanitarian Affairs (WFP)

***OHCHR** Office of the United Nations High Commissioner for Human Rights (also HCHR, UNHCHR)

OHRLLS Office of the High Representative for the Least Developed Countries, Landlocked Developing Countries and Small Island Developing States

OIE Office International des Epizooties (WOAH)

OMAEP World Organization for Parental Education Associations / Organisation mondiale des Associations pour l'Education parentale

OMCT Organisation mondiale contre la Torture / World Organization Against Torture / SOS Torture

***OPCAT** *Optional Protocol to the UN Convention Against Torture

OPCW Organization for the Prohibition of Chemical Weapons

OPEC Organization of Petroleum Exporting Countries

OPV Oral polio vaccine

OR Surgical: Operating room

ORS *Oral rehydration salts

ORSEC Disaster relief organization, France

OSCAL Office of the Special Coordinator for Africa and the Least Developed Countries/DESA

OSCAR Orbital Satellites Carrying Amateur Radio

OSCC On-site operations coordinating centre

OSCE Organization for Security and Cooperation in Europe

OSRO Office of Special Relief Operations

OST Office of Science and Technology (USA)
  *Outer Space Treaty

OVC Orphans and vulnerable children

OWRA Office of Weapons Removal and Abatement (USA)

OXFAM* *Oxford Committee for Famine Relief International

P

Pa *Pascal

PADCO Planning and Development Collaborative International

PAHO Pan American Health Organization *(WHO)

PAM Programme Alimentaire Mondial – *World Food Programme (UN)

Pap Medicine: vernacular abbreviation for Papanicolaou cervical test

PAR Population at risk

PASB Pan American Sanitary Bureau (PAHO)

PATH Programme for *Appropriate Technology in Health

PC Peace Corps

PCI Project Concern International

PCM *Protein-calorie malnutrition

PCNA Post-conflict needs assessment

PEC/WHO *Polio, Emergencies and Country Collaboration/WHO

PEM Protein-energy malnutrition

PEPFAR (USA) President's Emergency Plan for AIDS Relief

PERT Programme evaluation and review technique

PET Potential evapotranspiration Positron emission tomography

P4P Policy for planning

PFII Permanent Forum on Indigenous Issues

PHC *Primary health care

PHM *Prehospital medicine
  *People's Health Movement

PHR Physicians for Human Rights

PID Pelvic inflammatory disease

PIK Payment in kind

PIU Policy intelligence unit

PLS Prolonged life support (anaesthesia)

PMDF Proportion of maternal deaths among females of reproductive age

PMSC *Private military and security company

PNND Parliamentarians for Nuclear Non-Proliferation and Disarmament

PNP Private non-profit

p.o. Medicine: per os – by mouth

POMR Problem-oriented medical record

POP Fractures/orthopaedics: Plaster of Paris

POW *Prisoner of war or prisoner-of-war

PPE Personal protective equipment

PPH Post-partum haemorrhage *Pro-poor health strategy

PPM Public-private mix

PPP Purchasing power parity

PQMD Partnership for Quality Medical Donations

PRD/S Post-resuscitation disease/syndrome

***PRISM** *Prognostic risk of mortality

PROGRESA Programa de Educaciòn, Salud y Alimentaciòn

PRRO Protracted Relief and Recovery Operation (WFP)

PRS *Poverty reduction strategy

PSI *Population Services International

PSR Physicians for Social Responsibility

PTA Travel: prepaid ticket authorization Parent-Teacher Association

PTSS Programme and Technical Support Section (UNHCR) *Post-traumatic stress syndrome

PTWC Pacific *Tsunami Warning Center (Honolulu)

PUO Pyrexia (fever) of unknown origin

PVO(s) Private and voluntary organization(s)

Q

QAP Quick action project

Quake Vernacular abbreviation for earthquake

Quakers Friends World Committee for Consultation (Quakers)

QALE *Quality-adjusted life expectancy

QALY(s) *Quality-adjusted life year(s)

R

RA *Radium

RACES Radio Amateur Civil Engineering Service

***rad** Radiation absorbed dose (replaced by gray – Gy)

***Radar** Radio detection and ranging

RAMOS Reproductive age mortality studies

RAP *Rapid Assessment Protocol

R&D Research and development

RBC/rbc Medicine: red blood cells

RBM Roll Back *Malaria Partnership (WHO)

RC *Red Cross

RCPSC *Royal College of Physicians and Surgeons of Canada

RCRC *Red Cross and Red Crescent (ICRC)

RCT Randomized controlled trial

RDF Rapid Deployment Force (USA)

READI Euro-Arab Network of NGOs for Development and Integration

REC Regional Economic Community

Radda Barnen Swedish Save the Children Organization

Redd Barna Norwegian Save the Children Organization

*rem Roentgen equivalent man

REMPAN Radiation Emergency Medical Preparedness and Assistance Network

Res Rep Resident Representative (of UNDP)

R2P Right to *protection

Rh Medicine: Rhesus factor

RH Reproductive health

RHIB Rigid-hulled inflatable boat

RI *Refugees International

Ro-ro Roll on/roll off (ferry)

RT Register ton

RUTF Ready-to-use therapeutic food

S

s Second

S&T Science and technology / scientific and technological

SAA Small arms ammunition

SAAFA Special Arab Assistance Fund for Africa

SAARC Southern African Association for Regional Cooperation

SAB Skilled attendant at birth (as a proportion of total live births)

SADC Southern African Development Community

SAFE Surgery, antibiotics, facial cleanliness and environmental improvement

SAGE Strategic Advisory Group of Experts (on immunization),(WHO)

SAILD Service d'Appui aux Initiatives Locales de Développement

SALT *Strategic Arms Limitation Treaty

SAM Severe acute malnutrition Surface-to-air *missile

SAMU French EMS: Service d'Assistance Médicale d'Urgence

SAR *Search and rescue

SARAH Search and rescue and homing (radar system)

SAREC Swedish Agency for Research Cooperation with Developing Countries

SARS *Severe acute respiratory syndrome

SARSAT-COPAS Search and Rescue Satellite Aided Tracking

SATURN Specific Antibiotic Therapies on the prevalence of human host-resistant bacteria

SBA Standby arrangement(s)

SCF(I) Save the Children Fund (International)

SCHR Steering Committee for Humanitarian Response

Scuba Self-contained underwater breathing apparatus

SDC *Swiss Agency for Development and Cooperation

SDE Sustainable Development and Healthy Environments Cluster (WHO)

SDI *Strategic Defense Initiative ("Star Wars")

SDR Swiss Association for Aid to Developing Countries (SWISSAID)

SEA Sexual exploitation and abuse

SEARO Regional Office for South-East Asia (WHO)

SEATO South East Asia Treaty Organization

SEEHN South-Eastern Europe Health Network

SERPAJ Servicio Paz y Justicia (Uruguay)

SFB *Soya-fortified bulgur

SFCM *Soya-fortified cornmeal

SFP/C *Supplementary feeding programme / centre

SFSG *Soya-fortified sorghum grits

SGBV Sexual and gender-based violence

SHAPE Supreme Headquarters Allied Powers Europe (NATO)

SHARED Scientists for Health and Research for Development

SI Système International d'Unités (International System of Units)

SIAMED WHO model system for computer-assisted drug registration

SID *Society for International Development

SIDA Swedish International Development Authority

SIPRI Stockholm International Peace Research Institute

SITREP Situation report

SIW Self-inflicted wound

SKI Street Kids International (Canada)

SLBM Submarine-launched ballistic missile

SLCM Submarine-launched cruise missile

***SMS/GOES** Synchronous Meteorological Satellites / *Global-observing environmental satellites

SOLAS International Conference for the *Safety of Life at Sea

SONAR Sound navigation and ranging

SORT Strategic Offensive Reductions Treaty

SOS Save our souls (distress signal) *Surgeons OverSeas

SOST SOS *Torture

Soweto South-Western Townships (South Africa)

SP *The Sphere Project Samaritan's Purse

SPFS Special Programme for Food Security

SRAM Short-range attack missile

SRS Strategic rotating stockpile

SSSL Safe Surgery Saves Lives (WHO programme)

***START** *Strategic Arms Reduction Treaty
Simple treatment and rapid transport system

STD *Sexually transmitted disease(s)

SUMA Supply management for disaster relief (PAHO-WHO)

Sv *Sievert – unit of radiation dose

SWAps *Sector-wide approaches

SWAPO South West Africa People's Organization

SWEAT *Severe weather threat (WMO)

SWISSAID *Swiss association for aid to developing countries (SDC)

T

TA Transnational Authority

TAB Total absorbed dose (of radiation)

TAG Technical Advisory Group

TAT Toxin antitoxin

TB/Tb *Tuberculosis

TB/DOTS Directly observed treatment short course for tuberculosis

TBA *Traditional birth attendant

TBSA Total *body surface area (in burn injury)

TCAM *Traditional, complementary and alternative medicine

TCDC *Technical cooperation among developing countries

TdH Fédération Internationale Terre des Hommes

TDR Special Programme for Research and Training in Tropical Diseases (UNDP/WHO/World Bank)

TEKT *Technology enabled knowledge translation

Telex Teleprinter exchange

TF(s) Trust fund(s)

TFP/C *Therapeutic feeding programme/centre

TFR Total fertility rate

TI *Transparency International

TIR Transport International Routier/ International Road Transport

TISS Tata Institute of Social Sciences (India)

TMI *Three Mile Island (nuclear accident, USA)

TNM Tumour (size), node (involvement), metastasis (in cancer classification)

*TNT *2,4,6-Trinitrotoluene (chemical explosive)

TOKTEN Transfer of knowledge through expatriate nationals

TRC *Truth and Reconciliation Commission of South Africa

TRISS *Trauma and injury severity score

TS *Trauma score (AMA) Tidal scale

TSK Transitional shelter kit

U

U *Uranium

U3A University of the Third Age

UAM *Unaccompanied minor

UCI Universal child immunization

UER/EBU Union Européenne de Radiodiffusion / European Broadcasting Union

UFO Unidentified flying object

UHS Uncontrolled haemorrhagic shock

UHT Ultra-high heat treated (e.g. milk)

UMCOR United Methodist Committee on Relief

*UN *United Nations, United Nations Organization

UNA(s) United Nations Association(s)

UNAIDS United Nations Joint Programme on HIV/AIDS

UNCAC United Nations Convention Against *Corruption

UNCAST United Nations Conference on the Applications of Science and Technology

UNCCD United Nations Convention to Combat *Desertification

UNCED United Nations Conference on Environment and Development

UNCHR *United Nations Council on Human Rights (previously Commission)

UNCHS *United Nations Centre for Human Settlements – HABITAT

UNCIVPOL *United Nations Civil Police

UNCLOS United Nations Convention on the Law of the Sea

UNCT United Nations Country Team

UNCTAD United Nations Conference on Trade and Development

UNCSTD United Nations Conference on Science and Technology for Development

UNDAF United Nations Development Assistance Framework

UNDEF *United Nations Democracy Fund

UNDHR *Universal Declaration of Human Rights

UNDP *United Nations Development Programme

UNDPKO *United Nations Department of Peacekeeping Operations

UNDRO Office of the UN Disaster Relief Coordinator (superseded by *OCHA)

UNEP *United Nations Environment Programme

UNERC *United Nations Emergency Relief Coordinator

UNESCAP *UN Economic and Social Commission for Asia and the Pacific (also ESCAP)

*UNESCO *United Nations Educational, Scientific and Cultural Organization

UNFCCC *United Nations Framework Convention on Climate Change

UNFICYP United Nations Peacekeeping Force in Cyprus

UNFPA *United Nations Fund for Population Activities/UN Population Fund

UN-HABITAT *United Nations Centre for Human Settlements

UNHCHR *United Nations High Commissioner for Human Rights (also OHCHR)

UNHCR *United Nations High Commissioner for Refugees

UNHMH United Nations Humanitarian Mission in Haiti

UNHRD United Nations Humanitarian Response Depot (Brindisi)

UNIC(s) United Nations Information Centre(s)

UNICEF *United Nations Children's Fund

UNICRI United Nations Interregional Crime and Justice Research Institute

UNIDIR *United Nations Institute for Disarmament Research

UNIDO United Nations Industrial Development Organization

UNIFEM United Nations Development Fund for Women

UNIFIL United Nations Interim Force in Lebanon

UNIMAS United Nations *Mine Action Service

UNIPAC *UNICEF Procurement and Assembly Centre (Copenhagen *stockpile)

UNIRENE United Nations Informal Regional Network of NGOs

UNISDR *UN International Strategy for Disaster Reduction (OCHA)

UNITAID *UN International facility for purchase of diagnostics and drugs for tuberculosis, AIDS and malaria

UNITAR United Nations Institute for Training and Research

UNMIK United Nations Interim Administration Mission in Kosovo

UNODC *United Nations Office on Drugs and Crime

UNOG *United Nations Office at Geneva

UNON *United Nations Office at Nairobi

UNOOSA United Nations Office for Outer Space Affairs

UNOV *United Nations Office at Vienna

UNPFII United Nations Permanent Forum on Indigenous Issues

UNPROFOR United Nations Protection Force

UNRCA United Nations Registry of Conventional Arms

UNRISD United Nations Research Institute for Social Development

UNRWA *United Nations Relief and Works Agency for Palestine Refugees in the Near East

UNSCEAR *United Nations Scientific Committee on the Effects of Atomic Radiation

UNSCP United Nations Special Committee on Palestine

UNSECOORD UN Security Coordinator (New York)

UNSO *United Nations Sudano-Sahelian Office

UN-SPIDER United Nations Platform for Space-Based Information for Disaster Management and Emergency Response

UNU *United Nations University

UNV United Nations Volunteers

UNVFVT UN Voluntary Fund for Victims of Torture

UNW United Nations Women

UNWGIP UN Working Group on Indigenous Populations

UP United Press

UPI United Press International

URI/URTI Upper respiratory (tract) infection

USAID United States Agency for International Development (also AID)

UTC *Universal Time Consolidated

UXO/UXB Unexploded   ordnance/ unexploded bomb

UXOCE UXO Center of Excellence

V

VD *Venereal disease(s)

VDRL Venereal Disease Research Laboratory (for syphilis test)

VECTOR State Research Centre of Virology and Biotechnology (Russia, variola)

VHF Very high frequency (radio)

VITA Volunteers   in   Technical Assistance Inc.

VLBW Very low birth weight

VNGOC Vienna NGO Committee on Narcotic Drugs

VOICE Voluntary Organisations in Cooperation for Emergencies

VOLAG *Voluntary agency

VR Vital registration

W

W *Watt

WADEM *World Association for Disaster and Emergency Medicine

WAPS World Alliance for *Patient Safety (WHO)

WASH *Water, sanitation and hygiene

WBC White blood cells

WCC *World Council of Churches

WCED *World Commission on Environment and Development

WCRWC Women's Commission for Refugee Women and Children

WEFAX Weather facsimile communications system

WES Water and environmental sanitation

WFC World Food Council

WFH Weight for height (nutrition survey)

WFNS World Federation of Neurosurgical Societies

WFP *World Food Programme (UN)

WFSOS World Federation of Surgical Oncology Societies

WFSW World Federation of Scientific Workers

WHA *World Health Assembly (of WHO)

WHO *World Health Organization

WHODAS WHO Disability Assessment Schedule

*WHOPAX WHO Committee on the role of physicians in the preservation and promotion of peace

WIA Wounded in action

WIDER *World Institute for Development Economics Research (UNU)

WILPF Women's International League for Peace and Freedom

WINGS WFP Information Network and Global System

WIPO World Intellectual Property Organization (UN)

WJC World Jewish Congress

WLM Women's Liberation Movement

WMA *World Medical Association

WMD(s) *Weapon(s) of mass destruction

WMO *World Meteorological Organization (UN)

WOAH World Association for Animal Health (OIE)

WOAT World Organisation Against *Torture (SOS Torture)

WOFAPS World Federation of Associations of Paediatric Surgeons

WOH *World Open Hospital (*IAHM)

WOSM World Organization of the *Scout Movement (boy scouts/girl guides)

WPA World Psychiatric Association

WPC WHO Programme Coordinator

WPRO Regional Office for the Western Pacific (WHO)

WR *WHO representative
WRO (w.r.o.) (Commerce/insurance) war risks only
WSB *Wheat-soya blend
WSM *Wheat-soya milk
WSSD World Summit on *Sustainable Development
WTO World Trade Organization
WUS World University Service
WV *World Vision International
WWF *World Wide Fund for Nature International (formerly World Wildlife Fund)
WWSSN World-Wide Standard Seismography Network
WWW *World Weather Watch (WMO)
www World Wide Web

X

XDR Extensively drug-resistant disease

XDR-TB Tuberculosis caused by MDR strains also resistant to fluoroquinolone

Y

Y Young Men's/Women's Christian Association (formerly YMCA, YWCA)
YLDs Year(s) lost due to disability
YOB Year of birth
YPLL Year(s) of potential life lost

Z

ZEG Zero economic growth
ZMK Zentrum für Meeres- und Klimaforschung / Centre for Ocean and Climate Research, Germany
ZPG Zero population growth
ZT Zulu Time (see *Greenwich Mean Time)
ZZ *Zone zero